Getting What You Paid For:
Extending Medicare to
Eligible Beneficiaries in Mexico

**A research project directed by
David C. Warner**

A report based on research funded by
the Center for the Study of Western Hemispheric Trade
and the Hewlett Foundation

U.S.-Mexican Policy Report No. 10
Lyndon B. Johnson School of Public Affairs
The University of Texas at Austin
1999

© 1999 by the Board of Regents, The University of Texas System

Published in 1999 in the United States of America by the Lyndon B. Johnson School of Public Affairs, The University of Texas at Austin, Box Y, Austin TX 78713-8925

Book design: Doug Marshall, LBJ School Office of Publications

Getting What You Paid For: Extending Medicare to Eligible Beneficiaries in Mexico
Project Director: David C. Warner

ISBN 0-89940-329-8
Library of Congress Catalog Card No. 99-64677

This monograph is published under the auspices of the U.S.-Mexican Policy Studies Program at the Lyndon B. Johnson School of Public Affairs, The University of Texas at Austin. Established in 1988, the program promotes the study of significant policy issues affecting the United States and Mexico. Among these are research on U.S.-Mexican economic linkages, including the labor and environmental impacts of NAFTA; political decentralization in Mexico and its impact on the border region and on the binational relationship; and a variety of studies on the effects of trade, industrial regulation, health care delivery, migration, water management, transportation, and drug policy. The U.S.-Mexican Policy Studies Program and the reports are funded in part by a grant from The William and Flora Hewlett Foundation of Menlo Park, California. We gratefully acknowledge the support of the Hewlett Foundation in initiating this publication series.

U.S.-Mexican Policy Studies Program
Chandler Stolp, Director
Sidney Weintraub, Codirector

Policy Research Project Participants

Project Director
David C. Warner is a Professor of Public Affairs and holder of the Wilbur Cohen Professorship as a fellow at the Lyndon B. Johnson School of Public Affairs, The University of Texas at Austin. He has also been a visiting professor at The University of Texas School of Public Health since 1982. He teaches courses in economics, health care finance, and health policy and has published extensively on many aspects of health policy.

Contributors
Horacio G. Aldrete Sánchez has a B.A. in Public Accounting from the Universidad Autónoma de San Luis Potosí, Mexico. His interests are in public finance, regional development, and environmental issues.

Monica Clear has a B.A. in Political Science and Women's Studies from Rutgers. Her interests are in social services.

Susan M. Davenport has a diploma in nursing from St. Dominic's School of Nursing in Jackson, Mississippi, and a B.S. in Nursing from the University of Texas Medical Branch in Galveston. She has worked as a cardiovascular intensive care nurse and is interested in the medical legal field.

Olga Oralia Garcia has a B.A. in Public Policy from Occidental College. Her interests are in public health and issues affecting the elderly.

Anjum Khurshid has an M.A. in Economics and an M.B.B.S. (Doctor of Medicine) from The University of Punjab in Pakistan. He has served in the executive cadre of the civil service of Pakistan for eight years. His interests are in telemedicine, health care policy, and economic development.

Lauren Lacefield Lewis has a B.A. in Psychology from The University of Texas at Austin. Her interests are in public finance and information systems.

Dave Lawrence has a B.A. in Government from The University of Texas at Austin. He is currently employed as a Research Specialist at the Texas Department of Health. His interests are in international relations, defense policy, and health care policy.

Vanessa Catherine Murray has a B.A. in Anthropology from The University of Texas at Austin. She is currently employed as a Health Policy Associate with The Austin Project, a local nonprofit organization. Her interests are in health care and education policy, and science and technology issues.

Marissa Quezada has a B.A. in Sociology from Harvard College. Her interests are in health care policy.

Amy E. Sprague has a B.A. in Anthropology from the University of Notre Dame. Her interests are in international development.

Francie Kalunde Wambua has a B.A. in Legal Studies from The University of California at Berkeley. Her interests are in international and domestic economic development, environmental policy, and technology issues.

Ann Williams has a B.A. in Linguistics from Stanford University. Her interests are in international trade, business development, and innovative partnerships between the public and private sectors.

Contributing Editor

Lauren Rivera Jahnke has a B.A. in Biology from The University of Texas at Austin and an M.P.Aff. from the Lyndon B. Johnson School of Public Affairs, The University of Texas at Austin. She is currently a freelance policy researcher and analyst. Her interests are in health care policy, public health, and technology issues.

U.S.-Mexican Policy Studies Program Publications

Policy Report Series
Policy Report No. 1: *Free Trade with Mexico: What's in It for Texas?* (1992)

Policy Report No. 2: *Challenges in the Binational Management of Water Resourecs in the Rio Grande/Río Bravo* (1992)

Policy Report No. 3: *Policymaking, Politics, and Urban Governance in Chihuahua: The Experience of Recent Panista Governments* (1992)

Policy Report No. 4: *Health Care across the Border: The Experience of U.S. Citizens in Mexico* (1993)

Policy Report No. 5: *U.S.-Mexican Free Trade: The Effect on Textiles and Apparel, Petrochemicals, and Banking in Texas* (1993)

Policy Report No. 6: *Linking or Isolating Economies? A Look at Trucking along the Texas-Mexico Border* (1994)

Policy Report No. 7: *NAFTA and Trade in Medical Services between the U.S. and Mexico* (1997)

Policy Report No. 8: *Scarce Water: Doing More with Less in the Lower Rio Grande* (1998)

Policy Report No. 9: *New Federalism and State Government in Mexico: Bringing the States Back In* (1999)

Occasional Papers
No. 1: *Planning the Border's Future: The Mexican-U.S. Integrated Border Environmental Plan* (1992)

No. 2: *Australia and New Zealand: The Challenge of NAFTA* (1992)

No. 3: *Trade Liberalization in Mexico and the North American Free Trade Agreement* (1993)

No. 4: *Spatial Concentration and Efficiency in Mexican Industry: A Test of the Benefits versus the Costs* (1993)

No. 5: *The Evolving Protection of State Laws and the Environment: NAFTA from a Texas Perspective* (1994)

No. 6: *The Border Health Authority: Issues and Design* (1995)

No. 7: *Three Technical Papers on a Research and Demonstration Waiver for Medicare Coverage in Mexico* (1999)

No. 8: *Medicare Benefits for Recipients Living in Mexico: Proceedings of a Conference* (1999)

Other Publications

Texas-Mexico Transborder Transportation System: Regulatory and Infrastructure Obstacles to Free Trade (1991)

Maximizing Benefits of Tourism in Guerrero, Mexico (1991)

U.S.-Mexico Free Trade Agreement: Economic Impact on Texas (1992)

Sectoral Labor Effects of North American Free Trade (1993)

Aspectos económicos sobre transporte é infraestructura ante el reto del Tratado de Libre Comercio de América del Norte (in Spanish with executive summary in English) (1994)

NAFTA Handbook for Water Resource Managers and Engineers (1995)

The Impacts of Trade Agreements on State and Provincial Laws (1996)

For order information and book availability call 512/471-4218 or write to: Office of Publications, Lyndon B. Johnson School of Public Affairs, The University of Texas at Austin, Box Y, Austin, TX 78713-8925. Information is also available online at http://www.utexas.edu/lbj/pubs/.

Contents

Tables

Acronym List

AARP	American Association of Retired Persons
AARO	Association of American Residents Overseas
ACA	American Citizens Abroad
ACU	Ambulatory Care Unit
AMIS	Asociación Mexicana de Instituciones de Seguros (Mexican Association of Insurance Agencies)
ATM	Asynchronous Transfer Mode
BC/BS	Blue Cross/Blue Shield
CHAMPUS	Civilian Health and Medical Program of the Uniformed Services
CMPs	Competitive Medical Plans
DRG	Diagnosis Related Group
ECF	Extended Care Facility
ESRD	End-Stage Renal Disease
FFS	Fee for Service
FLAAG	Federated League of Americans Around the Globe
FMAP	Federal Medical Assistance Program
GDP	Gross Domestic Product
GFB	Grupo Financiero Bancomer (company name)
GME	Graduate Medical Education
HCFA	Health Care Financing Administration
HCPPs	Health Care Prepayment Plans
HCQIP	Health Care Quality Improvement Program
HMO	Health Maintenance Organization
HPSA	Health Professional Shortage Areas
IDS	Integrated Delivery System
IMSS	Instituto Mexicano de Seguro Social (Mexican Social Security Institute)
IPA	Independent Providers Association
ISDN	Integrated Services Digital Network
ISSSTE	Instituto de Seguridad y Servicio Social para los Trabajadores del Estado (Social Security for Mexican Government Employees)
JPEG	Joint Photographic Experts Group
LOS	Length of Stay
MCAT	Medical College Admission Test
MCO	Managed Care Organization
MCP	Monthly Capitation Payment
MFS	Medicare Fee Schedule
MSA	Medical Savings Account

NAFTA	North American Free Trade Agreement
NHIC	National Heritage Insurance Company
ORD	Office of Research and Demonstration (part of HCFA)
PCP	Primary Care Provider
POS	Point of Service option offered in some risk HMOs
POTS	Plain Old Telephone System
PPO	Preferred Provider Organization
PPS	Prospective Payment System
PRO	Peer Review Organization
RBRVS	Resource-Based Relative Value Scale
RVU	Relative Value Units
SNF	Skilled Nursing Facility
SSI	Supplemental Security Income
UNAM	Universidad Nacional Autónoma de México (National Autonomous University of Mexico)
UTHSC	University of Texas Health Sciences Center

Preface

THIS VOLUME IS THE RESULT OF A YEAR-LONG POLICY RESEARCH PROJECT AT the LBJ School of Public Affairs investigating the feasibility of extend ing Medicare coverage in some form to beneficiaries of the program who live in Mexico. This is the fourth in a series of research projects that have touched on this ongoing topic over the last nine years. The first project surveyed retirees in San Miguel, Guadalajara-Chapala, Mexico City, and Cuernavaca and also looked at hospitals and other facilities in these communities as well as surveying the literature on cross-border utilization. Our conclusion at that time was that such coverage would be advantageous to Americans living in Mexico and possibly could save the Medicare program funds as well.[1] Subsequent research related to this study included an examination of the ways in which the U.S. and Mexico could cooperate in providing health services in the future[2] and a study of NAFTA and trade in medical services between the U.S. and Mexico.[3] Although the second and third studies were somewhat tangential to the issue, one might legitimately ask why we have undertaken the current study.

The reason is simply that in spite of our conclusions eight years ago, there has been no appreciable movement toward examining the issue of Medicare coverage in Mexico. It has also become fairly clear that the Health Care Financing Administration (HCFA) would be unlikely to undertake such a significant change in coverage without a trial, such as a demonstration project. Because of the dispersed nature of the potential beneficiaries, their limited sophistication regarding reimbursement and health policy matters, and the lack of knowledge about the Mexican health system and U.S. retirees to Mexico in Washington, it has become clear that further investigation and fact-finding would be necessary to get this issue to the discussion stage. This report is the first part of that process. During 1998-1999, a second project will take place that will include a conference at which these findings and suggestions will be presented to an audience that will include retirees, health insurers, HCFA, providers, and other interested parties. Our goal with this project and the one to follow are to provide the background and to identify the relevant issues so that one or more demonstration projects can be initiated to test the impact of alternative changes in reimbursement policy.

Our ability to enter into this investigation has been enhanced by the support of the William and Flora Hewlett Foundation of the U.S.-Mexican Policy Studies Program at the LBJ School over the last nine years and also by the support provided by the Western Hemisphere Trade Center at the University of Texas and the LBJ School Policy Research Institute. The research has been the product of many students' hard work, motivated in part by the idea that this is a policy initiative whose time has come.

Notes

1. David C. Warner and Kevin Reed, *Health Care across the Border: The Experience of U.S. Citizens in Mexico,* U.S.-Mexican Policy Studies Program, policy report no. 4 (Austin, Tex.: Lyndon B. Johnson School of Public Affairs, The University of Texas at Austin, 1993).

2. Jeanette Hatcher, Jillian Hopewell, Adreana Guardiola, Kathy Jacquart, Walter Moreau, Jeffrey Stys, and David Warner, "The Border Health Authority: Issues and Design," U.S.-Mexican Policy Studies Program, occasional paper no. 6 (Austin, Tex.: Lyndon B. Johnson School of Public Affairs, The University of Texas at Austin, 1994).

3. David C. Warner, *NAFTA and Trade in Medical Services between the U.S. and Mexico,* U.S.-Mexican Policy Studies Program, policy report no. 7 (Austin, Tex.: Lyndon B. Johnson School of Public Affairs, The University of Texas at Austin, 1997).

Acknowledgments

THIS PROJECT WOULD NOT HAVE BEEN POSSIBLE WITHOUT THE HELP OF SEVeral experts and observers. Frances Ortiz Schultschik of Methodist Hospital in San Antonio and Pablo Schneider of Blue Cross/Blue Shield of Texas and Arizona deserve recognition for their assistance and guidance on various issues and requests as well as their willingness to visit the class. Special thanks to James Austin of MediPlan in Guadalajara, Ramon Baez of the School of Dentistry of the University of Texas Health Center in San Antonio, Kay Ghahremani of the Texas Health and Human Services Commission, and John Hilsabeck of the Texas Hospital Association for visiting with and speaking to our research group. Pedro Villarreal and Lucy Neighbors, staff members at the LBJ School of Public Affairs, greatly assisted in constructing the class Web page, arranging the research trips to Mexico, and offering overall support.

Anjum Khurshid served as a research assistant during the summer of 1997 (prior to the class), helping to gather background information and to identify resources and issues. He also compiled the various chapters into a single report and worked as a research assistant after the class in cleaning up the final document. Vanessa Murray formatted the feasibility survey, set up the database for survey entry, entered the surveys into the database, and compiled the analysis of the data. She also designed the class Web page and assisted in the editing and compilation of the final draft. David W. Lawrence graciously assisted in survey data entry and the data analysis. Amy Sprague compiled contact information necessary for future research. Ann Williams developed the name of the report. Lauren R. Jahnke served as the final editor and has substantially improved the final product. During this phase, Kevin C. Hendryx in the LBJ School Office of Publications served as the manuscript's copyeditor.

Chapter 4
Thanks go to Dr. Jorge Rodriguez Barrios at the Hospital de Nuestra Señora de la Salud, San Luis Potosí; Dr. Arturo Barrera at the Hospital de la Fe, San Miguel de Allende; Roger Allen at the American Legion, San Miguel de Allende; Louis and Paula Rosenblum of San Miguel de Allende; and Peter Oyler at *Atención San Miguel.*

Chapter 5
Thanks go to Baxter Brown and the staff of MediCasa; Norma Francis and the American Society in Guadalajara; and Adolf Horn of Bing's Ice Cream.

Chapter 6
Thanks go to Elaine Verdugo; Dr. Sergio Quintero Ruiz; Gloria Hernandez; Tilly Foster; Nova Sampieri; and Dr. J. Marco Capucetti and the staff at the Rosarito Family Care Clinic.

Chapter 10
Thanks go to Dr. Enrique Ruelas of Qualimed S.A.; Larry Meagher of the International Hospital Corporation; Pablo Schneider of Blue Cross/Blue Shield of Texas and Arizona; and Anna Marie Valle of the Universidad Ibero Americana de Tijuana.

Chapter 11
Thanks go to Javier Flores, Market Research Specialist of the United States Commercial Service, Mexico City; Actuary Eduardo Lara di Lauro, Managed Care Director of General de Seguros, Querétaro, Mexico; Dr. Casimiro Estrada Acuña, Medical Coordinator of General de Seguros, Hermosillo, Mexico; David S. Brown, Chief Operations Officer of Family Care Medical Systems, Livermore, California; Gustavo Novejas, General Director of Family Care Medical Systems, Chihuahua, Mexico; and Leticia Pérez Sanroman, Senior Trade Specialist, United States Embassy in Mexico, Mexico City.

Chapter 1
Introduction

by David Warner and Vanessa Murray

OVER THE NEXT THIRTY YEARS THE UNITED STATES MUST CONTINUE TO ADAPT to a world economy, further the process of integration of the nations of North America, and find equitable ways to reduce the high cost of a dependent aging population. One initiative which could help make progress in all three areas while also improving the lives of a number of elderly Americans would be to extend Medicare coverage to retirees in Mexico who are eligible for Medicare in the United States. Medicare, which accounted for $203 billion in expenditures in 1996, pays for most of the hospital and much of the physician expenditures of retirees.[1] U.S. retirees in Mexico number at least 100,000 and possibly more if all Medicare-eligible persons are counted. Even limited portability would be welcome to these beneficiaries, and would probably result in more persons choosing to retire to Mexico or to remain there after medical needs became greater. An evaluation of such portability will have to examine the cost and the quality of the care received as well as the ability of an entity to function as a fiscal intermediary for services delivered in Mexico. A demonstration project of coverage in Mexico could also serve as a model for more general portability of these benefits. As medicine is increasingly practiced through telemedicine and the Internet, limitations on coverage determined by place of residence should become less relevant.

Currently Medicare only pays for covered services outside the U.S. when a beneficiary is enroute to Alaska from the lower 48 states by a direct route or if a facility across the border is the closest for someone living or experiencing an emergency on the U.S. side. Medigap policies that do cover services abroad only do so for services to treat an emergency during the first 60 days of a trip. Since private coverage is not available to most applicants above a certain age from Mexican insurance companies, many retirees in Mexico are dependent upon the public system, if they enroll, or upon cash payments for care and the hope that they can get to the U.S. at an affordable cost if a major medical problem develops. In addition, Medicare beneficiaries have to make a decision regarding whether to enroll in Part B of Medicare and pay the monthly premium, which was $43.80 a month in 1997. For every year a beneficiary does not enroll in Part B, his or her subsequent premiums increase by 10 percent, and during that year the individual does not have coverage for physician's services, home health care, or other Part B services.

Retirees in Mexico are quite diverse in lifestyle, income, and degree of integration into Mexico. We conducted a nonrandomized survey of retirees in each of the three areas we studied during the fall of 1997 through spring 1998. The survey is reproduced in Appendix B and the responses are summarized in Appendixes C and D, as well as in relevant chapters. The vast majority of the retirees received Social Security and many had other sources of income. Most had obtained long-term residency papers in Mexico, and a majority of those responding had incomes below $25,000 a year, with almost a quarter having incomes below $15,000. Most gave cost of living and climate as their reasons for living in Mexico. Residents of all three areas would like to have Medicare cover services in Mexico. In a survey in 1990, 94 percent of those surveyed indicated they would seek medical services in Mexico if Medicare or veterans' benefits were available in Mexico.[2] Even many living in Ensenada or Rosarito find the 40-mile trip to San Diego onerous and expensive for routine medical care. Indeed, many of the retirees living in the trailer parks near these cities have very little financial margin and do not have the resources for such trips. They live where they do because they are able to live independently and near the ocean on very limited means. It is ironic that the entitlement that they have that is not means-determined (Medicare) is the one that is denied them, and because of that they may be forced to return to the U.S. and become dependent on means-tested aid.

Only in the Guadalajara-Chapala area did we find a number of retirees who bought into IMSS, the Mexican Social Security health system which covers nongovernmental employees of firms that pay into the system. Both Tricare, for military retirees and military dependents, and the Veterans Administration, for service-connected disabilities, reimburse beneficiaries for care received abroad. In fact, military retirees with CHAMPUS coverage who choose to live abroad face a problem when they turn 65. At that point, their CHAMPUS coverage is converted to Medicare coverage and they no longer have coverage abroad.

In addition to the three concentrations of U.S. retirees we studied, there are a number of persons who were born in Mexico who are eligible for Medicare and who have returned in retirement to their home towns or regions. Several of these individuals who we interviewed lived in small towns and had out-of-pocket expenses of US$300 to $600 a month. This was possible, in part, because they owned their own homes in these towns. In years to come, the number of Mexican-origin elderly in the U.S. is likely to grow significantly. Medicare coverage in Mexico would make retirement "back home" more attractive and, as with many of the U.S. retirees in the three areas we studied, permit an independent life free of the need to seek public help.

There are a number of policies short of total portability of all Medicare benefits reimbursed at full cost that should perhaps be considered as options. These include paying only for Part B services, paying for just Part A, or paying for emergency Part A services only. In each of these cases, reimbursement levels for comparable services could be substantially less than current Medicare reimbursement levels in the U.S. Another area that could be considered is limited reimbursement of long-term care by Medicaid using only federal funds for persons who have retired abroad. Finally, in a location like San Diego and northern Baja California, it might be possible to develop binational PPOs or HMOs that could enter into risk contracts to enroll residents of northern Baja who are Medicare beneficiaries. In fact, some of these arrangements might be partially accomplished with the Medicare Medical Savings Account option and some of the other options that may be available under the Balanced Budget Act of 1997.

The Health Care Financing Administration (HCFA) has a mandate to fund and evaluate research and demonstration waiver projects that have the promise of improving efficiency, beneficiary choice, and access for vulnerable populations. In general, these demonstrations have to show that they are at least revenue neutral. In addition, such a demonstration project would have to show that the quality of care was adequate, that administrative capacity was sufficient, and that beneficiaries were satisfied and believed themselves to be better off. In any case, several demonstration projects covering beneficiaries in Mexico would provide valuable information for future policy decisions as the U.S. and Mexican economies become further interdependent.

This book is organized into four sections. The first section, Chapters 2 and 3, describes the Medicare and Medicaid systems in the United States, including their benefit packages, financing mechanisms, and beneficiaries. Chapter 2 also includes a description of Tricare, the coverage available to military dependents and retirees that covers services in Mexico, as well as a discussion of some of the changes mandated by the 1997 Balanced Budget Act. Chapter 3 spells out a way in which Medicaid long-term care coverage could be federalized at fairly low cost for certain retirees in Mexico. The second section, Chapters 4 through 7, describes retirees in Mexico and the medical care system available to them in each of the three areas studied: San Miguel de Allende, Guadalajara-Chapala, and Ensenada-Rosarito-Tijuana. Chapter 7 looks at the potential growth of the Mexican-origin population in the United States and how coverage of services in Mexico might affect their retirement decisions. The third section, Chapters 8 and 9, presents several options for research and demonstration waiver projects including partial coverage and competing risk-based HMOs in northern Baja California. The final section, Chapters 10 through 12, examines some additional issues that should be considered in implementing coverage. Chapter 10 looks at the training of physicians in Mexico and quality assurance mechanisms which might be put in place. Chapter 11 surveys the development of private health insurance in Mexico and some current policy initiatives in Mexico that might enhance the role of private providers and insurers. Chapter 12 examines telemedicine, details how it has developed in Mexico, and speculates about how future arrangements between the U.S. and Mexico might work.

We hope that this report will demystify a number of topics. Furthermore, we hope that it will be used as a resource by those who seek to make the system of health care between these two countries more continuous and co-operative. And we hope that the decision to retire to Mexico will not continue to be made more expensive or impossible because of the nonportability of Medicare.

Notes

1. Katherine R. Levit, Helen C. Lazenby, Bradley R. Braden, and the National Health Accounts Team, "National Health Spending Trends in 1996," *Health Affairs,* vol. 17, no. 1 (Jan./Feb. 1998), pp. 35-51 (Exhibit 4: National Health Expenditures by Source of Funds, Amounts and Average Annual Growth, Selected Calendar Years 1960-96).

2. David Warner and Kevin Reed, *Health Care across the Border: The Experience of U.S. Citizens in Mexico,* U.S.-Mexican Policy Studies Program, policy report no. 4 (Austin, Tex.: Lyndon B. Johnson School of Public Affairs, The University of Texas at Austin, 1993), pp. 30-34.

Part 1
Medicare and Medicaid: Limitations on Coverage in Mexico

Chapter 2
Medicare Benefits and Waivers

by Anjum Khurshid and David W. Lawrence

T HE MEDICARE PROGRAM, AS ENACTED INTO LAW WITH THE PASSAGE OF THE Social Security Act, was designed primarily to provide health care cov erage for America's retirees. In the years that Medicare has been covering its beneficiaries, the health care industry has undergone many changes, ranging from increased use of technology in medicine to the emergence of health maintenance organizations (HMOs) and managed care. The general practitioner has been replaced by large medical complexes, medical specialists, and preferred provider organizations (PPOs). Consultations can be made from hundreds of miles away, and large health-providing conglomerates dominate the health services industry. Additionally, consumers are becoming more intelligent, more involved, and are making more informed decisions about their health care needs. The problem is that, with minor exceptions, Medicare currently does not cover services outside of the United States or its territories.

An understanding of the Medicare program and the benefits it provides is a crucial foundation to any examination of extending services to beneficiaries in a foreign country. The underlying purpose of this project is to determine if the need for such coverage exists, and if so, what would be the most appropriate mechanism for the provision of necessary services. This chapter explores various aspects of the Medicare program, new options for provision of health services implemented with the Balanced Budget Act of 1997, and other funding mechanisms for elderly and retired Americans. It concludes with a discussion of the use of research and demonstration waivers as a method of testing proposed changes to the Medicare program.

Medicare

The Medicare and Medicaid programs were established when Congress passed Title XVIII and Title XIX of the Social Security Act in 1965, and since that time these programs have been subject to numerous legislative and administrative changes. When Medicare started operating in 1966 it covered almost all persons over 65 years of age. However, later amendments have added other categories to the group of beneficiaries. In 1972, persons who are entitled to Social Security or Railroad Retirement disability benefits for 24 months or more and persons with end-stage renal disease (ESRD) requiring dialysis or renal transplant were added as Medicare beneficiaries. In 1973, elderly persons who were otherwise not authorized for Medicare benefits were allowed to pay a premium to become Medicare beneficiaries.

The Medicare program covers about 95 percent of the aged in the U.S. While total health care spending in the United States for calendar year 1996 was estimated at slightly over $1 trillion, Medicare alone was responsible for $203.1 billion.[1] The administrative costs for the program ranged from 1 percent for Part A to 2.6 percent for Part B. The combined Medicare benefit payments for all services in 1996 averaged $5,302 per enrollee. About 84 percent of the 38 million Medicare enrollees actually used the services in 1996.[2] Following is a summary of the main benefits provided by the Medicare program and the outline of the payment mechanisms employed by HCFA for these services.

Part A

Medicare consists of two main parts—Part A, or Hospital Insurance, and Part B, or Supplementary Medical Insurance. Eligibility for Part A is determined through the work experience of the beneficiary or the spouse (usually 40 quarters for those born after 1929). To buy into the system, the cost is determined by a formula derived by HCFA. For instance, with 30 to 39 quarters of coverage as defined by the Social Security Administration, the premium is $187 per month; for less than 30 quarters it increases to $311. In 1996, Part A provided coverage to about 38 million people, of whom 33 million were aged and 5 million were non-aged disabled beneficiaries. The benefits provided covered services worth $128.6 billion in 1996—an increase of 10.5 percent over 1995, with an average expenditure per enrollee of $3,400.[3]

Covered Services
- Inpatient hospital care (care received upon admission to a hospital)

- Inpatient care in a skilled nursing facility (following a hospital stay of at least three days, for patients recovering from illness or injury)

- Home health care (care in patients' homes)

- Hospice care (for terminally ill patients with life expectancy of six months or less who elect to forego traditional medical treatment for the terminal illness)

- Blood (blood processing, blood components, etc.)

Benefit Period

The benefit period starts when a beneficiary is admitted to a hospital and ends when the patient has been out of the hospital for 60 consecutive days. For each separate benefit period, beneficiaries have to pay an inpatient hospital deductible of $760 (in 1997). For this benefit period, Part A pays all the charges except the $760 deductible, but after 60 days of admission beneficiaries have to pay $190 per day up to day 90 (a practice known as "coinsurance"). Beyond 90 days, Part A does not pay anything except if the beneficiary uses the once-in-a-lifetime 60 Reserve Days benefit at a coinsurance rate of $380 per day.

There are four conditions for inpatient hospital care:

1. a doctor prescribes hospital care for treatment of illness or injury,

2. the type of care required can only be provided in a hospital,

3. the hospital participates in Medicare, and

4. the stay is not denied by a Peer Review Organization (PRO) or Medicare Intermediary.

In addition, Part A pays for all covered services for the first 20 days for a Skilled Nursing Facility (SNF), a limited number of visits for home health care, a maximum of 190 days in a lifetime for inpatient psychiatric care, and two 90-day periods of hospice care. There are no deductibles for hospice care, but for all other services the hospital submits bills to Medicare. Once Medicare approves the claim the bill is sent to the beneficiary for coinsurance and deductible payments.

Part A Payment

Medicare reimburses hospitals under Part A by the Prospective Payment System (PPS). There is a fixed payment based on Diagnosis Related Groups (DRGs). Payment is independent of length of stay or inpatient service, and is only based on the patient's diagnosis at the time of discharge. Hospitals must accept Medicare's payment as payment in full. Hospitals can, in extraordinary instances, be compensated for some of their excess costs for unusually costly services or long stays.

Skilled nursing facilities, hospices, and home health agencies are exempt from prospective payment and are paid under the reasonable cost method. Other types of hospitals with special rates include disproportionate share hospitals that serve a significantly disproportionate share of low income patients, sole community hospitals in rural areas that are the sole sources of care, and large teaching hospitals. Dialysis facilities, on the other hand, receive a set amount of payment per treatment called the composite rate, of which Medicare pays 80 percent ($139 in 1996).[4]

Claims Processing

HCFA contracts with various nongovernment organizations or agencies to serve as fiscal agents to process Medicare claims. For Part A services these agents are called fiscal intermediaries. These intermediaries process hospital insurance claims for institutional services, including claims from inpatient hospitals, skilled nursing facilities, home health agencies, and hospice services. The responsibilities of intermediaries include ensuring prompt payment to providers, establishing controls for utilization, keeping detailed records, performing regular reviews and audits of providers, determining costs and reimbursement amounts, and preventing fraud and abuse.

Part B

Part B, or Supplementary Medical Insurance, is available to almost all resident citizens age 65 and over. Part B coverage is optional and requires payment of a monthly premium. In Part B, federal general funds constitute about 75 percent of the costs and premiums make up the rest. In 1996 the program provided coverage to 36 million people and total benefits amounted to nearly $68.6 billion.[5] The program covers physician services (both hospital and nonhospital), clinical lab tests, durable medical equipment, diagnostic tests, ambulance services, and certain other miscellaneous services. Formerly, Home Health Agency services were covered in Part B only when there was no eligibility under Part A.

Part B Payment

Medicare pays for most Part B services using a Medicare Fee Schedule (MFS) derived by multiplying a national conversion factor, which is a dollar amount, by each procedure or service's relative value units (RVU), which reflect the resources involved in providing that procedure or service. Allowed charges for Part B are now either the lesser of the submitted charges or a fee schedule based on a Relative Value Scale. Durable equipment and clinical laboratory services are also based on a fee schedule. Outpatient services and Home Health Agencies are reimbursed on a reasonable-cost basis. Payment is adjusted by geographic areas. Medicare pays 80 percent of this payment for any service under Part B. Beneficiaries pay a 20 percent coinsurance copayment. The premium payment is $43.80 per month (in 1997), which is usually deducted from the monthly Social Security benefit check. Beneficiary premiums are currently set at a level that covers 25 percent of the average cost for aged beneficiaries.[6] Part B beneficiaries also had to pay an annual deductible of $100 in 1997 prior to receiving reimbursement for services.

Unlike Part A, providers under Part B are not required to participate in Medicare. Agreeing to participate in Medicare means that the physician requests direct payment from Medicare and that he/she agrees to accept Medicare's allowable as payment in full, regardless of actual charge. Electing not to participate means the physician has the choice on a claim-by-claim basis to accept "assignment." An assignment is an agreement between a physician and the insured where the insured transfers his rights to receive benefits to the physician, and, in return, the physician accepts Medicare's allowable payment as payment in full.

Unlike Part A coverage, if a person does not choose to pay the Part B premium he or she is not covered. A person with premium-free Part A benefits can sign up for Part B during a general enrollment period from January 1 through March 31 each year. Even if one lives abroad one must continue to pay for coverage. If one does not pay into Part B his or her subsequent premiums are increased by 10 percent for every year after age 65 for which a premium was not paid. This does not apply to those who are covered by their employer's or their spouse's employer's group health plan. A special enrollment plan is established for such people and they do not have to wait for the general enrollment plan. They may sign up for Part B during a special eight-month period, which is the eight months following termination of the employer's coverage.[7]

Claims Processing
Part B claims are handled by Medicare carriers. The responsibilities of the carriers are making payments to physicians and suppliers for services covered under Part B, determination of allowable charges under Medicare, maintaining quality of performance records, and preventing fraud and abuse.

Payment for Services Abroad

Medicare pays for health care in a qualified Canadian or Mexican hospital only under one of the following conditions:

- the beneficiary is in the United States when an emergency occurs and a Canadian or Mexican hospital is closer than the nearest U.S. hospital; or

- the beneficiary lives in the United States and a Canadian or Mexican hospital is closer to home than the nearest U.S. hospital (regardless of emergency or not); or

- the beneficiary is in Canada traveling by the most direct route between Alaska and another U.S. state and an emergency occurs that requires admittance to a Canadian hospital.[8]

Supplemental Health Insurance

Medicare does not cover all the health care services that a beneficiary might need. Some long-term care, most dental care, and outpatient pharmaceuticals, in particular, are not covered under Medicare. Insurance policies which fill these gaps in Medicare coverage are called Medigap policies. Both state and federal laws govern sales of Medigap insurance. Policies designed for this purpose must be specifically identified as Medicare supplemental policies. In addition, many Medicare recipients also have supplemental insurance provided to them by former employers as retirement benefits or they may also be covered by Medicaid, which covers many of these benefits.

Gaps in Medicare Coverage

The various gaps in coverage under Medicare that may be covered by supplemental health insurance include the inpatient hospital deductible for each benefit period ($760 in 1997), the $190 per day coinsurance for days 61 to 90 of hospital stays, all the costs after day 90 unless lifetime reserves are used, $380 per day coinsurance for each lifetime reserve day, coinsurance of $95 per day for days 21-100 in a Skilled Nursing Facility, and all charges after 100 days per benefit period. There are also gaps in Part B coverage, such as the annual deductible of $100 and coinsurance for 20 percent of Medicare-approved charges. There are other costs to the beneficiary as well, such as limited cost-sharing for outpatient drugs and inpatient respite care, and charges for the first three pints of blood.[9]

Current estimates are that Medicare pays only 45 percent of the total personal health care expenditures of people who are age 65 and older: 70 percent of hospital expenses, 61 percent of physicians' charges, 15 percent of other personal medical expenses, and 2 percent of nursing home costs. That is why most seniors (82 percent) have private coverage in addition to Medicare.[10]

Standardization of Medigap

During 1992 most states adopted regulations limiting the sale of Medigap insurance to no more than ten standard plans. These plans were developed by the National Association of Insurance Commissioners (NAIC) and were incorporated into state and federal law. The plans are designated with a letter from A to J, where A is the basic policy that all Medigap insurers must make available and J is the most comprehensive package, offering benefits that pay for services not fully covered by Medicare. The basic policy is available in all states and insurance companies are prohibited from changing the combination of benefits available by changing the letter designation. They are also required to use the same language, format, and definitions in describing the benefits of each Medigap plan. Table 2.1 shows the difference between different plans.

States can allow insurers to add "new and innovative" benefits to a plan that otherwise complies with applicable standards. The requirement for these benefits is that they should be cost-effective, not otherwise available in the marketplace, and offered in a manner consistent with the goal of simplification.

Open Enrollment

The open enrollment period for selecting Medigap policies guarantees that for a period of up to six months after the date a person is both age 65 and enrolled in Medicare Part B, he or she cannot be denied Medigap insurance or be charged a higher premium because of health problems. All standard Medigap policies are guaranteed renewable.[11]

Foreign Travel Emergency

Currently, supplemental health insurance Plans C through J provide for foreign travel emergencies. They pay for 80 percent of charges for emergency care received in a foreign country during the first 60 days of a trip outside the U.S. The beneficiary is responsible for a $250 deductible per calendar year. The lifetime maximum benefit is $50,000. This benefit fills the gap for travelers that is due to Medicare not covering care provided outside the United States except in limited circumstances.[12]

Medicare SELECT

In 1992 a new Medigap policy was introduced called Medicare SELECT whereby beneficiaries agree to use the services of certain hospitals and physicians (preferred providers) in return for lower premiums. Initially started in

Table 2.1
Medigap Plans and Benefits

	Plans									
	A	B	C	D	E	F	G	H	I	J
Basic Benefits	X	X	X	X	X	X	X	X	X	X
Skilled Nursing Coinsurance			X	X	X	X	X	X	X	X
Part A Deductible		X	X	X	X	X	X	X	X	X
Part B Deductible			X			X				X
Part B Excess						X	X		X	X
Foreign Travel Emergency			X	X	X	X	X	X	X	X
At-Home Recovery				X			X		X	X
Basic Drug Benefit								X	X	X
Preventive Care					X					X

Source: Health Care Financing Administration, "Types of Private Health Insurance," http://www.hcfa.gov/pubforms/98guide4.htm#Medigap. Accessed: November 17, 1998.

only 16 states, Medicare SELECT was expanded to all states in 1995 and authorized to continue until at least 1998 by Public Law 104-18, enacted by the 104th U.S. Congress to amend the 1990 Omnibus Reconciliation Act.[13] Under Medicare SELECT, when the beneficiary goes to a preferred provider Medicare pays its share of the approved charges and the insurer is responsible for the full supplemental benefits described in the policy.

Managed Care Plans
These are also called coordinated care plans, prepaid plans, or health maintenance organizations (HMOs). They cover the basic Part A and Part B package of benefits for a monthly premium but each plan has its own group of health care providers (physicians and hospitals) who offer medical services to members of a plan on a prepaid basis (capitation). Managed care plans enter into a contract with HCFA to provide Medicare-covered services to enrollees. HCFA pays the plan a monthly premium for each member, which is usually 95 percent of Medicare's average per capita cost of services in that county for a beneficiary with characteristics similar to the member. The advantage for members is that they do not have to pay the Medicare deductible and coinsurance for Medicare-covered services provided by the plan. Instead, the plan may charge a monthly premium or nominal copayments from the

beneficiaries. Beneficiaries still have to keep paying the Part B premium ($45.50 in 1999). Some managed care plans may provide additional benefits with little or no additional payment.[14]

There are three types of arrangements managed care plans might have under Medicare. The first are plans that agree to accept the financial risk of insuring and providing medical services for a Medicare beneficiary. They can require the enrollee to receive all covered care through the plan or through referral by the plan. If one gets services from providers outside the plan, neither the plan nor Medicare pays for these services. The only exceptions are emergencies received anywhere outside the service area in the United States. HMOs in some states must cover emergencies anywhere in the world.

The second type of plans base their contracts on the cost of services provided. They are not permitted to provide extra benefits at no cost and cannot require Medicare beneficiaries to buy extra benefits. Under these plans one can either go to the network of providers in the plan or one can go outside the plan. In the former case the beneficiary only pays the applicable copayment, while in the latter case Medicare pays its share of approved charges and the individual is responsible for the rest. Medicare reconciles actual allowable costs with the plan at the close of the enrollment period.

The third type of plans are similar to cost of service plans but may not provide all of the covered services under Medicare. These are called health care prepayment plans, or HCPPs. They are also not required to comply with all the conditions for the above two types; for example, HCPPs do not have to offer an open enrollment period.[15]

Tricare Standard Coverage

Tricare Standard (formerly CHAMPUS) is one of the Defense Department's regional managed health care programs for military retirees and dependents of active duty, retired, or deceased service personnel. This program covers military retirees who are not eligible for Medicare. Some U.S. citizens residing in Mexico are covered by Tricare Standard, and claims filed from Mexico are paid by Tricare similar to claims from within the United States. As one resident of San Miguel de Allende commented, "I have never understood why Medicare A and B are not available to U.S. residents in Mexico. CHAMPUS is able to provide reimbursement worldwide–why not Medicare?"[16] Wisconsin Physicians Service handles all foreign claims under Tricare and also those from Puerto Rico. A problem for people living abroad and covered under Tricare is that their coverage ends when they become eligible for Medicare Part A, which usually happens when the recipient turns 65.[17] Enrollees may continue to be eligible for Tricare after age 65 if Medicare issues a notice for disallowance that states that the enrollee did not work enough quarters in the United States to be eligible for Medicare coverage.[18] For this demonstration, it is valuable to examine the coverage Tricare Standard provides and how this coverage works in Mexico.

Tricare Standard pays a share of the cost of covered health care services for enrollees both in the United States and abroad. The enrollee is expected to receive care at a military hospital if one is available and if that hospital provides the kind of specific care the patient needs. If the hospital is within a 40-mile radius of the enrollee, it is considered to be available. Emergency situations, however, are exempt from this regulation.

Tricare Standard will also pay a share of the cost of covered health care from civilian providers. Covered health care includes emergency services and "medically necessary" services, including necessary inpatient services, outpatient visits, and institutional care such as mental health care and reha-bilitation. While Tricare Standard does not recommend a provider, it does maintain a network of providers. If the provider is within the Tricare net-work, then the patient is charged according to Tricare's standard charges. In addition, an enrollee of Tricare Standard may seek care from an authorized non-network civilian health care provider; however, Tricare pays claims based on its own list price.[19] If an out-of-network provider charges more than what Tricare allows for the claims, then the patient is responsible for the difference. Therefore, in general, using in-network providers results in less out-of-pocket expenses for the patient.

While not all services are covered, Tricare Standard does have set policies on paying claims. In all cases, there is no fee to enroll in Tricare Standard. The annual deductible is $150 for individuals or $300 for families. For covered outpatient, emergency, and mental health services from civilian provid-ers, Tricare Standard pays 75 percent of allowed charges. For covered civilian inpatient mental health services, Tricare pays the lesser of $137 per day or 25 percent of the institutional and professional charges. "Allowed charges" have been determined by Tricare Standard. It pays according to its allowed charges price list. If the charges exceed Tricare's price list–that is, if the provider is out of network–the patient is responsible for the difference. However, under U.S. law, providers are prohibited from charging more than 15 percent above Tricare's listed prices to Tricare patients.

Tricare Standard Overseas

General Procedures
Tricare Standard recognizes the needs of enrollees overseas. While many stan-dard domestic procedures apply to overseas patients, Tricare allows for cul-tural and logistical differences that may complicate health care services. As

with domestic procedures, the patient must go to a U.S. military hospital if one is available. If one is not available, the patient can choose a civilian provider. The patient pays the hospital and physician fees out-of-pocket and files a claim with Wisconsin Physicians Service. Tricare will reimburse the patient the percentage of allowable costs for each service rendered.

The Case of Mexico

In Mexico, the patient chooses where to seek health care since there are no U.S. military hospitals or network providers.[20] The patient pays the medical bills and files a Tricare Standard claim through Wisconsin Physicians Service. Tricare Standard reimburses the patient for 75 percent of covered, billed health care charges. The price list for domestic health care charges does not apply. Since the patient is free to choose the provider, there is no regulation of quality of care other than that the provider must be certified in his or her specialty. Researching providers and quality of care is left to the patient.

Tricare Standard does cover the cost of necessary medical evacuation from Mexico. However, Tricare Standard does not dictate to which U.S. hospital the patient will be transported. This coverage gives enrollees more flexibility with their health care, and the peace of mind to know that the care they need will be accessible in the event of an emergency.

The cost of extending Tricare Standard coverage to Mexico is relatively low. Regarding administrative costs, there is no Tricare Standard office in Mexico. As mentioned above, claims filed from abroad are handled though a branch of Wisconsin Physicians Service in Milwaukee. This office employs about 30 workers to cover all foreign claims, the majority of whom are claims processors and claims specialists.[21] Since care in Mexico is generally less expensive than care in the United States, Tricare pays less to a patient in Mexico than for a patient receiving similar care in the United States. A principal expense tied to extending Tricare to Mexico is issuing checks in Mexican pesos.

The office is sensitive to cases of fraud. Since claims in Mexico are much less expensive than claims in Mexico, acute cases of fraud are easy to detect. When claims filed from Mexico rival prices of those in the United States, then Tricare examines the claim for possible fraud. Instances are relatively low, but gross overcharges are obvious.[22]

In 1996 Tricare Standard received a total of 451 claims from Mexico. Of these claims, the government paid $655,071 and the beneficiaries covered $148,367. In 1997 the number of claims decreased dramatically, although the report for 1997 is not complete. (At the time of this writing, the report is estimated to account for 95 percent of claims.) In 1997 there was a total of 288 claims filed, costing the government $282,802 and the beneficiaries $69,686. While the number of claims decreased between 1996 and 1997, the number of claims from retirees stayed steady, with 125 retiree claims in 1996 and 109 in 1997. However, the costs paid by the government decreased from $332,612 in 1996 to $145,702 in 1997.[23] See Table 2.2 for a breakdown of claims and costs for 1996.

The Balanced Budget Act of 1997

The Balanced Budget Act of 1997 included important modifications to the Medicare program. These changes could have a significant impact on the feasibility of employing Medicare payments to provide health care for American retirees living outside the United States. Although no language was added or amended to explicitly include the provision of services to Americans residing in foreign lands, the changes may increase the likelihood of obtaining approval for a research and demonstration project from the Health Care Financing Administration (HCFA). Important changes resulting from the act are the creation of the Medicare Choice program and Medical Savings Accounts. In order to understand the changes enacted by the legislation, it is important to understand the procedures that existed prior to these amendments.

The decision to restructure the Medicare Risk HMO option was based on the limited success of the program. HCFA had not pushed this as an option, and thus it was a relatively unknown choice for most beneficiaries and not even available in most counties. HMOs were not available in many counties and others were unwilling to contract with HCFA for the available premium. In order to correct the shortcomings of the risk option, the Balanced Budget Act introduced the Medicare Choice option. The cost option is not affected by this legislation, nor is Medicare Choice designed to operate any differently than a traditional risk plan. The beneficiary contracts directly with an approved Medicare provider. Under Medicare Choice, several plans are available to recipients:

1. fee-for-service indemnity health plans that pay providers based on individually tailored health plans;

2. preferred provider organizations that offer beneficiaries the option of using providers who offer discounts;

3. provider-sponsored organization plans that are formed by affiliated providers and are paid at a capitated rate;

4. point-of-service plans that provide beneficiaries the option for using out-of-network providers (this option could be a model for a research and demonstration project that includes Medicaid);

Table 2.2
CHAMPUS Claims from Mexico and Costs, 1996 (in US $)

Type of Claim	Retirees (Average per capita cost)	Dependents of Retired/Deceased (Average per capita cost)	Dependents of Active Duty (Average per capita cost)	Combined (Average per capita cost)
Institutional				
Number of Claims	28	34	26	88
Government Cost	$145,922 ($5,212)	$103,454 ($3,043)	$62,649 ($2,410)	$312,026 ($3,546)
Patient Cost	$37,593 ($1,343)	$29,788 ($876)	$8,508 ($327)	$75,890 ($862)
Number of Admissions	22	25	17	64
Number of Days	268	177	43	488
Inpatient Professional				
Number of Claims	11	12	19	42
Government Cost	$56,855 ($5,169)	$5,757 ($480)	$26,742 ($1,407)	$89,356 ($2,128)
Patient Cost	$7,401 ($673)	$2,027 ($169)	$353 ($19)	$9,783 ($233)
Outpatient Professional				
Number of Claims	63	109	52	224
Government Cost	$126,602 ($2,010)	$97,602 ($895)	$17,815 ($343)	$244,021 ($1,089)
Patient Cost	$27,501 ($437)	$26,377 ($242)	$4,062 ($78)	$57,941 ($259)
Number of Services	1,816	2,040	311	4,167
Pharmacy				
Number of Claims	23	57	17	97
Government Cost	$1,231 ($54)	$5,510 ($97)	$2,925 ($172)	$9,667 ($100)
Patient Cost	$1,708 ($74)	$2,192 ($38)	$850 ($50)	$4,751 ($49)
Grand Total				
Number of Claims	125	212	114	451
Government Cost	$332,612 ($2,661)	$212,325 ($1,002)	$110,134 ($966)	$655,071 ($1,452)
Patient Cost	$74,205 ($594)	$60,386 ($285)	$13,775 ($121)	$148,367 ($329)

Source: Wisconsin Physicians Service, "Champus Foreign Country Report for Care Received in Fiscal Year 1996–Mexico" (printout from Wisconsin Physicians Service, Madison, Wisconsin), 1996, n.p.

5. health maintenance organizations that operate as traditional HMOs and pay for services at a capitated rate;

6. Medical Savings Accounts (MSAs), which will be discussed in greater detail; and

7. any other plan that suits the needs of the beneficiary and is offered by a HCFA-approved contractor.[24]

As with previous Medicare HMOs, a person is eligible if they are entitled to Medicare Part A and enrolled in Part B, except if he or she has already been diagnosed with end-stage renal disease. Again, like the Medicare HMO option, a person diagnosed with renal failure after enrolling in the Medicare Choice program is eligible to remain in the plan. Medicare Choice plans are responsible for offering open enrollment periods during the month of November, when plans expire, and also when new beneficiaries become eligible. Enrollees are automatically renewed in the program and cannot be dropped from their plans, except in case of fraud or nonpayment. Beneficiaries may, however, leave plans at any time to enroll in other Medicare Choice options or choose a traditional Medicare option.[25]

Under the umbrella of Medicare Choice plans is the Medical Savings Account (MSA). This account is a discretionary pool of funds available to the individual recipient for payment of qualified medical expenses. Federal regulations have not yet been written for MSAs, but the way MSAs are planned to operate is that Medicare recipients may choose to establish an MSA as their Medicare Choice plan. The recipient will enroll in a health insurance policy from an approved provider that carries a high deductible and covers both Parts A and B. (The deductible must be between $1,500 and $2,250 for 1999.) HCFA will pay the deductible of the insurance policy and make annual contributions into the individual's MSA equal to the difference between the premium for the insurance policy and the Medicare Choice capitation rate in the beneficiary's county. Deposits into the MSA will not be considered taxable income, and withdrawals from the account that are used for medical expenses are also not considered as taxable income. If funds are not used for qualified medical purposes during that year, the withdrawn funds are treated as taxable income while the retained funds accrue interest tax free. MSAs are designed to provide the same options that private insurance policyholders enjoy, and the high deductible is designed to prevent frivolous use of benefits.

The Medical Savings Account provides the consumer the flexibility for self-determination of what medical procedures and expenses are necessary. The MSA demonstration offers one of the more promising opportunities for coverage in Mexico. If this is truly discretionary money, then it should be up to the beneficiary to determine how and where services are rendered. However, until the specific regulations are delineated in the Code of Federal Regulations, the criteria for utilization of MSA funds are uncertain.

Waivers

In order to adapt successfully to the rapidly changing environment in which health care is provided, HCFA employs various mechanisms to assess the conditions of the health care market and determine what changes are needed to make both Medicare and Medicaid more efficient and effective programs. The waiver is one such instrument of modification.

Waivers allow HCFA to amend specific policies and allow programs to operate in the manner most appropriate for given situations. Typically, three types of waivers are issued by HCFA. Section 1915(c), Section 1915(b), and Section 1115 waivers each are used to modify certain aspects of HCFA's programs. The 1915(c) waiver is a specific Medicaid waiver designed to offer states the flexibility to develop and implement alternatives for providing services for eligible individuals who would otherwise be in facilities such as nursing homes. The 1915(c) waiver is referred to as the "home and community-based" waiver. The 1915(b) is the "freedom of choice" waiver, also specific to Medicaid, and it is designed to improve beneficiary access to care through enrollment in a guaranteed provider network. In particular, it offers a choice of providers in areas where Medicaid managed care is being implemented while permitting the state to restrict choice to several approved plans rather than all licensed providers. Both the 1915(c) and (b) waivers have time limits on their initial duration and are renewable. The home and community-based waiver has a duration of three years and is renewable every five years, and the freedom of choice waiver has a two year duration and is renewable every two years.

The 1115 "research and demonstration" waiver is a more generic waiver that applies to Medicaid, Medicare, and other Social Security Act programs. Unlike the Medicaid program waivers, the 1115 waiver does not have the constraints associated with the 1915(c) and (b) waivers. Demonstration waivers can be requested to custom fit programs to specific areas, allow certain specific services, or modify other structural aspects of programs. The important requirement that HCFA places on demonstration waivers is that they be budget neutral, that is, that they generate no additional cost over what HCFA would normally spend. These waivers are usually five-year projects, after which an evaluation of their success is completed.[26]

The HCFA Office of Research and Demonstrations (ORD) is the entity that conducts Section 1115 demonstrations and is ultimately responsible for their evaluation. The range of activities under the ORD includes examination of delivery of services, adequacy of services, beneficiaries and their needs, providers, contractors, and just about any other variable in HCFA's arena. The ORD conducts these demonstrations and evaluations with their own staff as well as awarding grants and contracts to separate entities to conduct research.

Currently, the ORD has four primary themes for research and demonstration projects aimed at providing better services to HCFA's customers. The first theme is the monitoring and evaluation of health system performance through the criteria of access, quality, efficiency, and cost.[27] Under this theme, public programs are studied regarding program efficiency and utilization, and tools are developed to enhance the capacity of the ORD to conduct research in this area. The Medicare and Medicaid programs are systematically scrutinized in order to determine if any changes need to be made. The conclusions from this research are then considered for formal demonstration projects. In order to support this theme, the ORD established the following objectives:

- produce descriptive statistics on the health system's infrastructure;

- produce descriptive statistics on populations of heath care users;

- develop monitoring and evaluation tools to support evaluation of HCFA programs;

- evaluate differences in access to care;

- evaluate the impact of managed care on access to care, health care costs, and quality of care;

- evaluate the effects of HCFA programs on beneficiary health status; and

- monitor fraud and abuse and program integrity.[28]

The second theme is improving health care financing and delivery mechanisms. Under this theme, the ORD seeks to improve current methods of health care financing and develop new payment, cost containment, and financing systems for HCFA's programs. This theme requires research and demonstration projects to explore alternatives to the fee-for-service system and to focus on the beneficiary with respect to streamlining the administration and focusing on needs. Objectives include

- developing new payment, quality assurance, and delivery systems for acute care, post-acute care, and long-term care;

- developing new approaches for managing high-cost and high-risk patients;

- developing new delivery models for managed care;

- developing models of beneficiary-directed care;

- developing improved risk adjustment mechanisms for payments to managed care organizations; and

- developing other innovative delivery and payment models.[29]

The third theme evaluates meeting the needs of vulnerable populations. This group of vulnerable peoples includes minorities, the frail elderly, women with high-risk pregnancies, and underserved populations such as inner-city urbanites, rural inhabitants, migrant workers, refugees, and the disabled. Objectives include extending benefits to new populations, developing new payment and delivery systems that integrate acute and long-term care, understanding and improving long-term care financing, and developing new payment and delivery models for health care in rural areas.[30]

The fourth theme is gathering information to improve consumer choice and health status. Data regarding preferences and needs of consumers is a prerequisite to implementing policies designed to improve accessibility and affordability. HCFA also needs to know how healthy various populations are before new initiatives can be implemented. Research and demonstration projects under this theme are designed to gather and process the necessary types of data. Objectives established include producing information to assist providers and beneficiaries in assessing medical treatment options, producing information to assist beneficiaries in choice of health care plans, and providing information to improve beneficiaries' health status.[31]

The underlying purpose of this policy report is to propose options for the extension of Medicare, or aspects of it, to Mexico. Knowledge of waivers and waiver processes is essential in order to know what procedures must be followed to test the idea or ideas through the waiver process. Knowledge of Medicare and other Social Security Act provisions is essential in order to know what requirements or restrictions need to be waived. The combination of these different and often dynamic pieces needs to come together in such a manner that Medicare can be made to fit within the Mexican health care network and American retirees living in Mexico can utilize Medicare benefits. Waivers are the logical first step to the ultimate implementation of Medicare in Mexico.

Notes

1. Katherine R. Levit, Helen C. Lazenby, Bradley R. Braden, and the National Health Accounts Team, "National Health Spending Trends in 1996," *Health Affairs,* vol. 17, no. 1 (Jan./Feb. 1998), p. 36.

2. Health Care Financing Administration (HCFA), "Brief Summaries of Medicare and Medicaid," http://www.hcfa.gov/medicare/ormedmed.htm. Accessed: February 23, 1998.

3. Ibid.

4. HCFA, "Medicare Kidney Coverage," http://www.medicare.gov/publications/kidney.pdf. Accessed: November 17, 1998.

5. HCFA, "Brief Summaries of Medicare and Medicaid."

6. Ibid.

7. Office of Federal Register, National Archives and Records Administration, Code of Federal Regulations, Title 42, Public Health, Parts 400-429 (Washington, D.C.: Government Printing Office, 1991).

8. HCFA, "Medicare Part B Coverage," http://www.medicare.gov/publications/mhbkc03.htm. Accessed: November 17, 1998.

9. HCFA, "1997 Guide to Health Insurance for People with Medicare," http://www.hcfa.gov/medicare/97guide2.htm. Accessed: March 4, 1998.

10. Health Insurance Association of America (HIAA), "Issue: Medicare Supplement Insurance," http://www.hiaa.org/consumerinfo/medicare.html. Accessed: April 6, 1998.

11. HCFA, "Types of Private Health Insurance," http://www.hcfa.gov/pubforms/98guide4.htm#Medigap. Accessed: November 17, 1998.

12. Ibid.

13. HCFA, "1997 Guide to Health Insurance for People with Medicare."

14. HCFA, "Managed Care/Medicare Plus Choice Manual," http://www.hcfa.gov/pubforms/mcmpcm/c00.htm. Accessed: December 1, 1998.

15. Ibid.

16. Comment received on survey from a respondent in San Miguel de Allende, LBJ School Survey of U.S. Retirees in Mexico, 1998.

17. Department of Defense, *Tricare Standard Handbook* (Aurora, Colo.: Tricare Support Office, 1997), p. 8.

18. Ibid., p. 30

19. Ibid., p. 5.

20. Karen Piraino, Tricare Standard, "Tricare in Mexico," Personal email to Amy Sprague, March 5, 1998.

21. Telephone interview by Amy Sprague with unidentified claims processor, Wisconsin Physicians Service, Madison, Wisconsin, March 23, 1998.

22. Ibid.

23. Wisconsin Physicians Service, "Champus Foreign Country Report for Care Received in Fiscal Year 1997–Mexico" (printout from Wisconsin Physicians Service, Madison, Wisconsin), 1997, n.p.

24. HCFA, "Medicare+Choice Part C Statuatory Requirements and Regulatory Implementation," http://www.hcfa.gov/medicare/medicare/mplusc.htm. Accessed: February 3, 1998.

25. Ibid.

26. HCFA, "Medicaid Waivers," http://www.hcfa.gov/medicaid/obs7.htm. Accessed: September 16, 1997.

27. HCFA, "Research and Demonstrations," http://www.hcfa.gov/ord/ordhp1.htm. Accessed: February 26, 1998.

28. Ibid.

29. Ibid.

30. Ibid.

31. Ibid.

Chapter 3
Medicaid Extended to Mexico

by Lauren Lacefield Lewis and Marissa Quezada

T HIS CHAPTER WILL PROVIDE A BRIEF INTRODUCTION TO MEDICAID. PRIMA-rily, we will examine issues for the aged and disabled who are eligible for Medicaid, how the basics of the Medicaid system in the U.S. work, and how we may be able to help some of the aged and disabled get the health care support they need in Mexico.

First, we will examine issues for Medicaid-eligible persons, including the difficulty of maintaining a decent standard of living in the United States on a limited income and the potential advantages available to those wishing to relocate to Mexico. Second, we will look briefly at how the federal Medicaid system works to support people in the U.S. through community-based services and institutional care such as nursing facilities. Third, we will look at the possibility of making health care support available to aged and disabled recipients of Medicaid in Mexico: specifically, we will examine the services available, possible means of reimbursement, and other important considerations in funding health care services in Mexico. Finally, we will look briefly at the possibility of reducing Medicaid dependency for some aged and disabled Medicaid recipients.

Background

There is significant concern over the ability of the U.S. government to provide the financing necessary to keep pace with the increasing level of health care need in this country. In fiscal year 1997, HCFA reported spending $160 billion on Medicaid alone.[1] This concern is shared by both the federal government and state governments who contribute funds toward this program. As a result, new legislation is supporting increased options and experimentation to controls costs and to provide more access to high-quality services.

However, it is not only the government that is concerned about making ends meet. Most Medicaid recipients in the U.S. are struggling to maintain a minimum standard of living and get the care that they need to stay independent. The income allowed to Medicaid recipients does not allow most persons to live well in the United States but would be sufficient for a significantly higher standard of living in Mexico.

The notion of allowing elderly and disabled persons with Medicaid the freedom to move to Mexico and utilize Mexican health care resources may be one way to meet the needs of both governmental entities and retired persons. Section 1915(c) of the Social Security Act is a means of accomplishing this. Section 1915(c) allows states to establish programs to provide services at home or through the community rather than at medical institutions such as nursing homes.[2] In this chapter, the notion of community-based services offered to Medicaid recipients in Mexico will be examined. In addition, we will look at some of the issues raised by the possibility of having the entire cost of the program paid for by HCFA out of their minimum federal contribution to Medicaid costs.

What we are proposing is not an entitlement to Medicaid services for all aged and disabled persons residing in Mexico, but a useful option that may make sense for some people living on a limited income.

Issues for the Aged and Disabled

What Is It Like to Live in the U.S. on Medicaid?

Medicaid recipients are allowed different incomes in different states. However, in general there are established allowed incomes based on a given percentage of federal income poverty limits. In Texas, the *Medicaid Provider Manual for Long Term Care Facilities,* Section 4100, states that clients on Supplemental Security Income (SSI) are automatically financially eligible to enter a long-term care facility under Medicaid. Clients above the SSI limits but below $1,482 per month in income must first be certified by Medicaid Eligibility (ME) staff at the Texas Department of Human Services.[3]

Furthermore, Congress has enacted a law that requires states to protect the income and assets of spouses of Medicaid-eligible persons by allowing them to retain $1,357 per month (as of July 1998), and states may further extend this benefit range to $2,019 per month. States must also allow the spouse to retain the greater of $16,152 in assets or half the couple's joint assets up to $80,760.[4] *Spousal impoverishment* is a Medicaid provision whereby the resources and income of a spouse are partially protected when the other spouse is institutionalized. However, most spouses of Medicaid beneficiaries do not have nearly this much to keep.

What Would It Be Like to Live in Mexico with that Amount of Support?

We interviewed residents of large cities like Guadalajara and found that many people were living very comfortably on only US$600 or $700 per month.[5] The people we spoke with had one- or two-bedroom apartments in good neighborhoods with parks and corner stores for only US$250 per month. They indicated that they spend another 400 or so dollars on food, entertainment, and basic living expenses. Some even indicated that they traveled back to the U.S. once or twice a year, took regular one- to three-day excursions around Mexico, and visited the opera and ballet. Moreover, many persons have cut expenses by not owning a personal vehicle. In Guadalajara, there is excellent public transport which allows many retirees to get around the city without the cost of maintaining a personal vehicle. Persons who live in smaller communities may find that public buses are not readily available; however, even in these areas there may be taxis for inexpensive transportation.

Why Doesn't Everyone Go to Mexico?

Although many find moving to Mexico an ideal alternative to living in poverty or near-poverty in the United States, many retirees point out that one of the keys to living successfully in another country is feeling that you have a choice in moving. Many retirees tell stories of people who felt angry that they would have such a poor standard of living in the United States. Some of these people either have difficulty adjusting to their new environment or choose to return to the United States.[6] Others find that they miss families, churches, and familiar friends and neighborhoods too much to leave them permanently. Some families miss the presence of grandparents in the lives of their children when the retirees leave for another country. Another major barrier seems to be arranging for reasonable quality health care in Mexico. Today, although most of these persons paid into the Social Security system their entire working lives and continue to pay income tax to the U.S. government, they cannot utilize the plentiful and affordable high-quality health care in their communities in Mexico. While their Mexican neighbors receive house calls and benefit from personal relationships with their doctors, U.S. citizens often travel back and forth from Mexico to get care until they are no longer physically able to travel and are forced to move to nursing facilities and high-cost, long-term care in the United States. The retirees we spoke to felt that this was what was most difficult about their situation: they had made good friends and new homes for themselves that they would ultimately have to leave so that they could get the affordable medical care they need.[7]

Why should the Government "Allow" People the Freedom to Relocate in Mexico?

In response to rising costs and the desire for more individualized health and personal care support services, the U.S. health care system is in transition from an institutional to a home- and community-based service system. In general, this is a more cost-effective and desirable system for receiving care. As the Baby Boomers age, there are significant concerns that the government will no longer be able to finance basic health care for all seniors. Pilot projects have been undertaken nationwide to try to find options that expand choices for Medicaid recipients, make better quality care available, and increase financial efficiency. In particular, attempts to provide both Medicare and Medicaid in a coordinated way have been pursued.

These two trends are very much in line with the idea behind this proposed pilot program. Medical care in Mexico is highly community based: doctors make house calls, nurses can be hired out to provide services in the home, and live-in domestic help is very affordable. This home-based system has developed, one may argue, because institutional care is not usually an option for Mexicans with elderly family members. Since many women do not work outside the home, they are the ones who usually undertake the task of caring for their parents even in times of extended illness. Another reason institutional care is not considered even when families have the financial ability to provide it is because putting one's parent(s) in a home is often seen as culturally inappropriate in Mexican society.[8] Moreover, medical costs in Mexico are significantly cheaper than in the United States. This creates an opportunity for persons who choose to live in Mexico and utilize these services to effect a cost savings for the U.S. government. Most retirees living in Mexico consider this a win-win situation.

The Basics of the Medicaid System

Medicaid is a joint program (state and federally funded) created by Title XIX of the Social Security Act to provide medical assistance for the indigent. Although each state can have its own definition of indigency, there are broad federal income limits regarding who is eligible for Medicaid funds. Title XIX requires that in order to receive federal matching funds, certain basic services must be offered to the categorically needy population in any state program. The most important services are listed below:

- inpatient hospital services;

- outpatient hospital services;

- physician services;

- medical, surgical, and dental services;

- nursing facility services for individuals age 21 or older;

- home health care for persons eligible for nursing facility services;

- rural health clinic services and any other ambulatory services offered by a rural health clinic that are otherwise covered under a state plan;

- laboratory and X-ray services;

- family nurse practitioner services; and

- federally qualified health center services and any other ambulatory services offered by a federally qualified health center that are otherwise covered under a state plan.

States may also receive federal funding if they elect to provide other optional services. The most commonly covered optional services under the Medicaid program include the following:

- clinic services;

- optometrist services and eyeglasses;

- prescribed drugs;

- TB-related services for TB-infected persons;

- prosthetic devices;

- dental services; and

- Intermediate Care Facility Services.

States may provide home and community-based care waiver services to certain individuals who are eligible for Medicaid. The services to be provided to these persons may include case management, personal care services, respite care services, adult day health services, homemaker/home health aide, habilitation, and other services requested by the state and approved by HCFA.[9]

The portion of the Medicaid program that is paid by the federal government, known as the Federal Medical Assistance Program (FMAP), is determined annually for each state by a formula that compares the state's average per capita income level with the national average. By law, the FMAP cannot be lower than 50 percent nor greater than 83 percent. Wealthier states such as Connecticut and New Hampshire receive 50 percent, while Mississippi currently receives 77 percent. Texas received 63 percent in FY 1997. The federal government also shares in the states' expenditures for administration of the Medicaid program. Most administrative costs are matched at 50 percent for all states. However, higher matching rates (75, 90, and 100 percent) are authorized by law for certain functions and activities.[10]

Generally, persons living on SSI or on Social Security and making no more than approximately $1,500 per month from all sources with no large cash reserves are financially eligible for Medicaid-funded institutional care and many home and community-based programs throughout the country. Specifics vary from state to state, with some states only allowing applicants who meet SSI criteria to be eligible for the aforementioned programs.[11] In addition, each person must be judged eligible by age or disability. Periodic re-evaluation of clients' financial eligibility for Medicaid is necessary for both long-term care facilities and general eligibility.[12]

In order to receive services, each Medicaid recipient must also have a determination as to whether his medical needs meet certain established criteria. For high-cost care such as nursing facility placement, this decision (called Medical Necessity) is made in Texas by the Utilization Review Committee of National Heritage Insurance Company (NHIC) (Section 4810). In different states, different requirements apply. For example, in Texas a recipient must only have difficulty with one Activity of Daily Living, while in some other states three activities must be adversely affected.[13]

Each state makes payments to vendors according to a predetermined schedule. Many make payments to long-term facilities on a monthly basis and reimburse other providers on a fee-for-service basis. In order to receive timely payments, providers must have specific forms properly filled out in order to receive payment authorization.[14]

Each state determines guidelines for providers with regard to making records available for review by staff of the individual states and other state organizations with a regulatory or fraud-deterrent function. For example, in Texas, Medicaid providers must make records available for review by the Texas Department of Human Services (TDHS) and the Attorney General's Medicaid Fraud Control Unit at any time. Clinical records of former patients must be retained for five years after medical service ends.[15] Each contracted provider must submit financial and statistical information to the state annually in accordance with all pertinent published cost-reporting rules and report instructions.[16]

Home Health Agencies and other providers across the country undergo a process for licensure, certification, and renewal. The purpose of licensure is to protect the public by ensuring the existence of an adequate level of desirable services for public use. Licensure inspections confirm that acceptable care is being provided and that state and local building and fire codes are met. Surveys for licensure compliance are conducted during the licensing period.[17]

Each state is responsible for auditing nursing facilities and other care providers to verify compliance with the requirements and contractual agreements. Each state is also responsible for investigating all reports of abuse and neglect occurring in their long-term care facilities. Criminal liability exists if any nursing facility employee fails to report known abuses.[18]

Waiver Exceptions

Several conditions of participation would have to be modified or waived by HCFA in order to cover care in Mexico. Some of these are quality of life, licensing, nurse assistant competency and evaluation, and residency requirements. In light of the reduced reimbursement proposal, it would seem reasonable to allow Mexican home health agencies to meet different standards than those presently imposed in the U.S. Similarly, some of the licensing conditions of participation could not be met in Mexico, as many of these conditions are tied to U.S. regulators' inspections and staffing requirements.[19]

Providing Health Care Support in Mexico

Nursing Facilities and Community Care in Mexico

There are few services in the cities of Guadalajara and San Miguel de Allende that could fit the bill of a typical nursing facility in the U.S. There are not many nursing facilities elsewhere in Mexico, for that matter, as most Mexican families prefer to care for their elderly at home. The main type of nursing facility available in Mexico is called *sala general* (general room). This is basically a large room with many elderly persons sleeping in it. Most of these are run by Catholic organizations in Mexico and are for the truly destitute who would otherwise be dead or living on the street. These organizations do not provide even basics such as blankets, soap, prescription medicines, or nursing care. The families provide these if possible; otherwise patients may do without. The costs for these are approximately N$500 monthly (approximately US$60).[20]

In Guadalajara there are no acceptable nursing facilities available comparable to American facilities, but there is one in the Lake Ajijic area called Casa Nostra. Even at this seemingly high-quality facility, families must arrange for doctors, nurses, appropriate forms of therapy, and necessary prescriptions for their loved ones. It should also be noted that this trend toward home-based care may change over time, and "American-style" nursing facilities may eventually appear in Mexico. An advantage to the current dearth of nursing facilities is that it would be much easier for Mexico to go straight to community-based services. The problem with this is that community-based programs are generally administered by home care agencies.

There is an emerging agency in Guadalajara called MediCasa that is very reputable, but as of yet it has no planned date to expand to the San Miguel de Allende area. Once home health agencies become more commonplace in Mexico, community-based programs could expand into San Miguel and other areas. A community-based project may need to be piloted in Guadalajara initially, since this is the only regional location that has a viable home health agency which could likely offer all the integral services of a community-based program.

Models for Payment

In this section we will discuss the implications of expanding Medicaid coverage by using one of three different models of community living available in the United States: a provider-based program, direct financial support, and a managed care program for community-based services. In addition, we will discuss possibilities for funding nursing facility care in Mexico.

Each model will be based on the same general idea of creating a system that is dependent on federal funds only. We are proposing that each person who signs up for this program be eligible to receive one-half of the federal percentage that Medicaid would pay in a more affluent state. In other words, the federal government would pay 25 percent of the average cost of the service in the U.S. The client could then receive services according to the model he or she selects.

Provider-Based Program in Community Living

This program would design a plan of support and provide the care that is needed through a single care organization and supplemental contracts handled by the central agency. Individuals and families may have input into the choice of providers, but these providers are employees of or consultants to a provider agency.

In the United States, case management is provided for by an agency that is separate from the service provider. This model focuses on client independence and the integration of the client into everyday community life. Services include case management, habilitation, respite care, nursing services, psychological services, physical therapy, occupational therapy, speech pathology, adaptive aids/supplies, and minor home modifications.[21]

Services would be provided by a home health agency, temporary staffing service, or a clinic or hospital that provides home-based care. Case coordination would need to be provided by a separate organization. Since social workers are less of a presence in Mexico, there is not a clear choice for selecting an organization to support these professionals.

One possible means of administering such a program would be through a U.S.-owned intermediary who reimburses both the case management entity and the direct care agency (which would probably be a home health care agency). It would be important that the intermediary have the ability to reimburse care providers soon after services are rendered. A 72-hour turnaround time would help alleviate the tendency of providers in Mexico to raise rates for those payers whose reimbursements take a substantial period of time. This is a legitimate concern in Mexico, where inflation rates can rise rapidly and currency exchange risks are substantial. With all of these things in mind, reimbursement rates should be substantially lower for equivalent services in Mexico. However, a provider-based program tends to be a more expensive model for services. This is primarily due to costs to the provider organization to recruit, hire, train, and schedule support staff. In other models, such as the direct monetary support model, many of these tasks are taken on by family members.

Direct Monetary Support

This program would grant benefits to individuals with physical disabilities to purchase services that would enable them to live in the community. Eligible individuals can choose and purchase an array of goods and services.

Program participants may purchase or lease special equipment or make architectural modifications to a home to facilitate the care, treatment therapy, or general living conditions of a person with a disability. In addition, they may purchase medical, surgical, therapeutic, diagnostic, and other health services related to a person's disability. When needed, program participants may utilize counseling and training programs that help provide complete care for an individual with a disability.

Many program participants utilize attendant care, home health services, home health aide services, homemaker services, and chore services. In addition, the program covers respite care, transportation services, and preapproved transportation and room and board costs incurred by the disabled person or his family during evaluation or treatment. Finally, many other disability-related services are available with prior approval by the appropriate state entity.

What we are proposing in this project transforms this program very little. In the United States the caseworker assists the client in securing care providers according to an agreed-upon plan of care. In Mexico the client would need additional assistance in locating appropriate services and may need reimbursement for some extraordinary expenses such as translation services, but other than that, this program is designed to be highly flexible and to meet the needs of individuals in very different communities.

One possible means of administration would be through a U.S.-owned intermediary who approves a plan of care and performs some monitoring through local case management services of the care and services purchased with these dollars. This model would reimburse both the case management entity and provide direct payments in one lump sum or in several installments (as appropriate). Since beneficiaries would receive payment from HCFA in advance of services being provided, any home health care services, supplies, or other support services could be paid for at the time the services are rendered. This would be especially helpful in that individuals could negotiate their own fees with providers (which tend to be less than when large foreign organizations negotiate a rate) and providers could be paid immediately, as is the custom throughout Mexico. Reimbursement rates should be substantially lower for equivalent services in Mexico. Direct payment programs in the U.S. tend to be extremely cost-effective as well as flexible in the ways that they meet the needs of individuals. Based on the interviews with local retirees, many individuals have the ability to determine their support needs, seek in-home assistance, and coordinate their own care. This type of model is ideal for many who are able to hire and schedule the support staff they need to stay independent.

The three different models for reimbursement have different levels of expense associated with their operations. The cheapest to operate would be a direct payment option where the family or individual takes on many tasks. For this reason, the amount of dollars available to individuals who enroll in these plans where they must take a more active role and where the administration costs are decreased as well should be somewhat greater than the plans where either an HMO or provider organization takes on this role for substantial fees.

Managed Care Option

Using a comprehensive care approach, this program provides an array of services for a capitated monthly fee that is below the cost of comparable institutional care. Covered services include any and all health-related services including inpatient and outpatient medical care, specialty services like dentistry and podiatry, social services, in-home care, meals, transportation, day activity, and housing assistance.

It would be possible to create a program based on a managed care model that offers services on both sides of the U.S.-Mexico border. It could also be operated as a managed care option with all but the most exceptional technical care provided in Mexico. (In practice, by the time that the elderly would qualify for this option, most would be unable or unwilling to travel to the United States even for specialty care.) This would necessitate bringing some services up in standards or assuring a relatively comparable service. In addition, it would mean bringing together a network of providers that may include psychologists, psychiatrists, and specialized therapists in addition to a traditional network of physicians.

One possible means of administering this would be through a U.S.-owned intermediary who reimburses a local managed care entity in Mexico. It would be important that the intermediary have the ability to provide sufficient funding to the HMO so that it can reimburse care providers within a very brief time frame from the time that services are rendered. As mentioned previously, a 72-hour turnaround time would help alleviate the tendency of providers in Mexico to raise rates for those payers whose reimbursements take a substantial period of time.

Reimbursement rates should be substantially lower for equivalent services in Mexico. The HMO model should be somewhat cheaper than the provider-based model and may provide greater accountability and efficiency. However, it could be significantly more costly than a direct payment model. It should be noted that an HMO model in Mexico should still be substantially less expensive than an equivalent model in the United States.

Nursing Facilities

If it were decided to fund nursing facilities in Mexico, there could be several different options for Medicaid reimbursement to providers of care for the retired population residing in Mexico. HCFA could use a direct payment model where the enrollee is directly paid 25 percent of the average cost of the service if it were received in the United States. The client could then administer the money in the fashion he or she desires. The client's family would choose the appropriate nursing facility (and any supplemental medical costs in that facility) in Mexico and pay the providers' fees. The family would also hire the nurses and doctors who were eligible to receive Medicaid payment and buy needed prescriptions with this amount. This type of system would benefit from good oversight activities to prevent misappropriation of dollars and assuring recoupment when appropriate.

Another method would be to have a third party administer the program in Mexico, most likely through a well-established insurance company in Mexico such as Seguros Monterrey Aetna or Comercial América. If this were the case they would have to follow the Medicaid system of coding and reimbursement. Due to the likelihood of fraud in this area it would be necessary to maintain close supervision of the administrators in Mexico. It must also be noted that unlike in the U.S., payments for those in nursing facilities would regularly have to be rendered to other sources such as pharmacies, doctors, and nurses, as these services are not included in Mexican nursing facilities' fees today. Mexican HMOs would potentially be the most preferred provider of services in today's health care climate. However, there is only one viable HMO-like organization in all Mexico today (Guadalajara's MediPlan). The development of other HMOs in Mexico will most likely occur in the next few years and could help Medicaid administer the project.

Considerations and Concerns

In attempting to transport these community-based services to Mexico there will be some common issues despite different modes of delivery. These include eligibility, service availability, continuity of care, special provisions to avoid abuse and neglect, and additional services needed when operating in foreign countries.

There are some overall issues to be addressed in considering support for persons with disabilities who move with a caretaker to Mexico. First, one should consider continuity of care. There is a basic question as to what will happen if the caretaker becomes incapacitated or dies. Second, it is important to maximize choices. There is a major concern that an aged person or one with a disability will become isolated by language, unable to find employment, have difficulty socializing with same-age peers, or have difficulty locating specialized professional support and consultation when needed. Third, one would want to avoid forced relocation. What will stop providers in the U.S. from forcibly relocating persons with disabilities to Mexico as a cost-saving measure? What real choice does a person with a disability have if their foster care provider decides to relocate to Mexico? Fourth, there is a possibility of relocation by choice. What if a person with a disability decides to live independently in Mexico? Or wishes to move to the home or facility of a Mexican national? These are all questions that would have to be answered in a good community-based waiver that includes both the aged and the disabled.

Eligibility

In the United States, eligibility for community-based services is built upon having a level of need that would qualify an individual for nursing facility care. For these persons, one must opt out of facility-based care for community-based care. In nursing facilities, eligibility is based upon having an income within specified limits and having the need for assistance in activities of daily living. The allowable income and the number of daily living skills that must be impaired differs from state to state.

Eligibility standards in Mexico should be able to remain consistent with current standards other than the provision that a residence be maintained in the United States. It may be appropriate to have an option for portable coverage. For example, some individuals may wish to move back and forth between the U.S. and Mexico. These program participants should be able to maintain coverage. One of the biggest questions is whether individuals will be able to receive coverage in any area of Mexico or only in certain regions. If individuals can settle anywhere in the county, there would have to be a complete set of intermediaries, trained service providers, and an ability to conduct evaluation and follow-up activities across Mexico.

A large problem with eligibility determination would be the occurrences of eligibility fraud in Mexico. In the U.S. there are currently mechanisms in place in order to lessen fraud in reporting resources and income. The Internal Revenue Service reports to individual state Medicaid offices income received by Medicaid clients reported to them by employers and (more pertinent with an elderly population) amounts of interest that were on IRS Form 1099. From there one can infer how much was in a savings account, especially if the amounts of interest earned are sizable. For Medicaid recipients in the U.S. it is easy for those with connections to Mexico to hide assets today. A reliable branch/branches of the Office of Inspector General must be established in order to help reduce the amount of fraud that could occur.

Quality Assurance
Clients would have the right to appeal any decisions rendered by the eligibility specialists as they do today. They would have 90 days to appeal any denial or reduction of benefits.

Peer Review
Peer review is a concept that is standard in the United States among health care professionals and is growing in favor in Mexico today. A form of this must take place in Mexican nursing facilities as well as with community-based providers in order for quality to improve to near U.S.-accepted levels of care. This could be done by regional provider groups in Guadalajara and San Miguel de Allende/San Luis Potosí.

Continuity of Care Issues
Continuity of care can be difficult to achieve in the United States even with its plethora of resources, established organizations, and trained social workers. A plan to make support services available to the aged and disabled in Mexico must have a clear plan to assure continuous support services, excellent monitoring, and emergency coverage. This is one reason that it would be helpful to have case management and services occurring through different organizations to provide some basic checks and balances. In addition, monitoring and reporting requirements may need to be increased somewhat to assure continuous provision of services.

Licensing and Inspection
One of the most obvious difficulties of reimbursing for care in Mexico is the

distance issue. Conducting even routine inspections of nursing facilities and providers in Mexico would be much more difficult. In addition, there are many legal considerations; for example, jurisdiction would have to be determined with local health authorities regarding investigations of professional misconduct.

Special Provisions to Avoid Abuse and Neglect

In Mexico, formal reporting of abuse and neglect is not consistently practiced. In addition, there are not clear repercussions for unprofessional or abusive behavior. It will be important that guidelines and standards are clearly outlined, effectively communicated, and that follow-up education and support activities are maintained for professionals who are taking on these new roles and expectations. Finally, although there are standards in the U.S., it will be important to organize them in a way that is as consistent as possible with existing guidelines for professional conduct that are already present in Mexico.

A private U.S. carrier, such as Blue Cross, might be a reasonable choice for assuming the role of coordinating investigations of misconduct in Mexico. The carrier could conduct reviews of Medical Necessity and other eligibility determination. This eligibility determination could be done by phone and paper, as it is now at many state Medicaid offices. Face-to-face interviews are rarely employed today as the primary interviewing method. One would probably have to extend the time frame for completion of cases from 90 to 180 or more days, as the time-lag with mail to Mexico would be a formidable barrier. A U.S. carrier would probably be more appropriate than a Mexican government entity because it would be held accountable for problems and would assume a limited form of liability, while a government agency within Mexico (such as Secretaría de Salud) would not.

Additional Services Available to Support Living Abroad

In order to provide quality services in Mexico, it is important to include some services that are not covered in the United States. Some initial services which should be considered include the education of physicians and other service providers regarding guidelines, expectations, best practices, and other skills and knowledge necessary to provide requested support services in Mexico. In addition, a significant amount of translation services may be required, especially in regard to consultation from specialized therapists and acquiring medical/therapeutic supplies from local providers. Finally, services like telemedicine and other consultation from U.S.-based specialists should be reimbursed to assure not only immediate coverage for requested services, but development of skills and knowledge by local professionals and other caregivers.

Goods and Services Availability in Mexico

Some services that are necessary in a high-quality waiver may not be available in all parts of Mexico; some are not available even in the largest cities. For example, occupational therapists and occupational health nurses are not available even in large cities like Guadalajara. Furthermore, it is not clear whether specialists in seating and positioning or speech therapists will soon be widely available. In addition, specialized medical equipment in Mexico tends to be costly and out-of-date. This would be especially problematic for persons with physical disabilities who require wheelchairs with seating systems that are frequently adjusted and who need bed and bath lifts.

Case management is a service that may be difficult to develop in Mexico. Because social workers are not the strong presence that they are in the United States, some basic activities such as discharge planning and home health care are rare. There may be a great deal of education that would need to be done in order to provide this service. Case managers will be of particular importance since they are in many ways a "gatekeeper" and responsible for primary quality assurance activities.

If adult foster care remains an available service, this project must answer the question of whether only U.S. nationals would be eligible to serve as foster families. Even if it were decided that only U.S. nationals could serve as foster families, these persons would need respite that is often provided by friends, neighbors, or semiskilled professionals on a short-term basis. There is always a possibility that in the event of the illness or incapacitation of a foster family, a client would choose to relocate temporarily or full-time with their respite provider.

Quality assisted living and residential care services are difficult and costly to operate on a small scale. These more structured living environments may be better provided through more intensive home support services through a home health agency. In addition, participants who propose minor home modifications will probably benefit with more stringent guidelines than are currently required for modifications that occur in the United States, to assure compliance with appropriate safety specifications.

One advantage to living in Mexico for program participants would be the abundance of individuals who are potential personal assistants and/or respite providers. Assuming that there are sufficient professionals in the region to provide some basic orientation and training for these workers, it will not be difficult to find good quality assistance with participants' basic living needs.

Finally, HCFA would need to give careful consideration to fair ratesetting and allowable services in Mexico. Because the health care system is very different in Mexico, there may need to be some limitations on approved providers due to the wide variety of education and skill as well as use of modern technology. It is important that the government and retirees both receive the highest quality care and services possible while in Mexico.

Other Aspects

Other aspects of patient care could be addressed by having either written or oral surveys taken by a neutral party in Mexico. The results could then be forwarded to HCFA and/or the insurance company responsible for payment to the nursing facilities or CBA (Community-Based Alternatives) providers. Poor results, along with problems uncovered by audits, could be grounds for termination of a Medicaid contract.

A Federally Based Medicaid Program

The proposed project of providing some support for Medicaid beneficiaries in Mexico offers a unique opportunity. Because the costs to provide medical care in Mexico are so much less than in the United States, it is felt that appropriate coverage could be provided with only a portion of the federal minimum contribution. This would mean that instead of each state adopting its own version of these proposed models and seeking approval from HCFA, it would be possible to have a program which is consistent throughout the United States for all its citizens.

Consistency between states is especially helpful for programs such as this where the beneficiaries are coming from across the United States. Since any individual state may not have a large number of retirees in Mexico, it would be helpful to have all the administration done together in order to achieve efficiencies of scale and better measurement of outcomes for the project. However, current law requires a state, in partnership with HCFA, to petition for a waiver of certain requirements in Medicaid regulations in order to provide a new or innovative program under the research and demonstration project. Since no state would be asked to make a contribution, the question arises as to why we would need to develop a separate plan in each state, especially if there does not seem to be a substantial benefit from doing so.

Whether each state would need to develop its own plan, managed separately, or whether the federal government could sponsor this project directly will have a major impact on the direction of this project. This will be a serious question that must be addressed prior to substantial work on a potential Medicaid waiver of the sort described in this chapter.

Notes

1. Interview by Lauren Lacefield Lewis with Dick Ladd, former Commissioner, Texas Health and Human Services Commission, Austin, Texas, March 30, 1998.

2. U.S. Congress, House Committee on Commerce and Subcommittee on Health and the Environment, testimony by Sally K. Richardson, Director of Medicaid Bureau, Health Care Financing Administration (HCFA), June 22, 1995.

3. Texas Department of Human Services (TDHS), *Medicaid Eligibility Handbook,* Section 1000 (Austin, Tex., October 1997), p. 13.

4. Health Care Financing Administration (HCFA), "Spousal Impoverishment," http://www.hcfa.gov/medicaid/obs10.htm. Accessed: January 10, 1998.

5. Interviews by Lauren Lacefield Lewis with anonymous retirees, Guadalajara, Mexico, March 15, 1998.

6. Ibid., March 17, 1998.

7. Ibid.

8. Interview by Marissa Quezada with anonymous retirees, Ensenada, Mexico, December 14, 1997.

9. HCFA, "Overview of the Medicaid Program: Medicaid Services," http://www.hcfa.gov/medicaid/mservice.htm. Accessed: January 10, 1998.

10. Ibid.

11. Ibid.

12. TDHS, *Medicaid Eligibility Handbook,* Section 1100, p. 15.

13. Ladd interview.

14. HCFA, "Overview of the Medicaid Program: Payment Procedures," http://www.hcfa.gov/medicare/ormedmed.htm. Accessed: January 10, 1998.

15. TDHS, *Medicaid Provider Manual for Long Term Care Facilities,* Section 4150 (Austin, Tex., October 1997), p. 81.

16. HCFA, "Overview of the Medicaid Program: Cost Reporting," http://www.hcfa.gov/medicaid/crmedmed.htm. Accessed: January 10, 1998.

17. HCFA, "Overview of the Medicaid Program: Home Health Agencies and Primary Home Care," http://www.hcfa.gov/medicaid/hhmedmed.htm. Accessed: January 10, 1998.

18. HCFA, "Overview of the Medicaid Program: Program Financing and Vendor Liabilities," http://www.hcfa.gov/medicaid/pfmedmed.htm. Accessed: January 10, 1998.

19. David C. Warner, *NAFTA and Trade in Medical Services between the U.S. and Mexico,*

U.S.-Mexican Policy Studies Program, policy report no. 7 (Austin, Tex.: Lyndon B. Johnson School of Public Affairs, The University of Texas at Austin, 1997), p. 339.

20. Interview by Marissa Quezada with Enfermera Luisa Solon, Asilo de Ancianos, Tijuana, Mexico, October 14, 1997.

21. HCFA, "Overview of the Medicaid Program: Medicaid Services."

Part 2
Medicare Beneficiaries in Mexico: Case Studies

Chapter 4
San Miguel de Allende

by Horacio Aldrete and Amy Sprague

S AN MIGUEL DE ALLENDE IS A CHARMING COLONIAL TOWN THAT LIES IN A mountain valley in the state of Guanajuato, Mexico, 170 miles north west of Mexico City. Due mainly to its year-round agreeable climate, quaint atmosphere, and relatively inexpensive cost of living, San Miguel has become a haven for American retirees. With a total population of close to 80,000 inhabitants, San Miguel is home to approximately 3,500 U.S. citizens.[1] The Americans that live and work in San Miguel de Allende constitute a well-organized and active community. With their participation in varied activities ranging from painting to providing Internet services, they play an important role in San Miguel's economic development.

Population

The U.S. citizens residing in San Miguel are a diverse population. Not only do their interests vary, but they also vary greatly in their economic circumstances. Many have moved to San Miguel specifically for the opportunity to live better than they could in the United States since they are able to take advantage of the lower cost of living in Mexico, regardless of their economic levels. Our survey results show that 75 percent of respondents in San Miguel specifically cited the cost of living as a main reason why they moved to San Miguel (see Appendix C: Data by Question, Question 26).

The residents in San Miguel have settled in a variety of ways regarding housing and amount of time spent in Mexico each year. Some have bought homes, ranging in size from modest to rather large. Others have opted to buy plots and build the houses themselves. Still others prefer to rent and take advantage of relatively low rental prices. Renters include those who have recently moved to San Miguel and who are looking for a home to buy. In addition, many renters comprise the group of U.S. citizens that live in San Miguel part-time, which according to our survey results constitutes approximately one-third of the U.S. population in San Miguel. Many of these part-time residents find it easier to rent while living in San Miguel. Other part-time San Miguel residents prefer to own a house and rent it to other part-time U.S. residents. These partnerships tend to work favorably for both parties, since both can enjoy part-time living in San Miguel relatively cheaply. In addition, while there is relatively little apartment housing, some U.S. residents choose to live in a type of group home; for example, some members of the Lion's Club may board at the club.

Other U.S. citizens have moved to San Miguel because they enjoy the culture. Regardless of the primary reason for moving to Mexico, all have noted the cheaper way of life Mexico provides. Many of those who are living with meager means often cannot afford a trip to the United States for necessary health care to take advantage of their Medicare benefits. Our survey results show that residents in the lower income brackets would be more willing to seek health care in Mexico if it were covered under Medicare. Residents in higher income brackets who might be able to afford a return trip to the U.S. may prefer not to return for routine care; however, they are also more likely to seek care in the U.S. even if Medicare covered services in Mexico. Furthermore, those in the higher income brackets are probably more likely to travel frequently to the U.S. anyway, and naturally they would be more likely to seek health care in the U.S. Regardless of income brackets, several retirees in San Miguel have stated that at least they would like the option to use Medicare in Mexico. One retiree commented, "Medicare should cover retirees wherever we go. It is insupportable that so many Americans live at least part-time in Mexico and our medical insurance ends at the border." Another said, "I think many U.S. citizens would welcome the acceptance of Medicare in Mexican hospitals and prefer to be treated in Mexico[2]

According to our survey, almost 20 percent of those who have returned to the U.S. for health care in the last three years have cited affordability as their primary reason to return to the U.S. (see Appendix C: Data by Question, Question 8.) Several others specifically cited that they returned to the U.S. to be covered under Medicare. Others sought health care in the U.S. because they were already in the U.S. visiting relatives or friends, or on business. Since they are not covered in Mexico, it was easier for them to seek health care while they were in the U.S. The Americans we surveyed agreed, independent of their economic status, that Medicare coverage in Mexico would save both themselves and Social Security a lot of money.

With almost all the U.S. residents in San Miguel at or approaching retirement, most are eligible for Medicare benefits in the United States. They either travel back to the U.S. for health care, buy insurance to cover Mexican health care, or pay for each medical visit or procedure directly out-of-pocket, which is the most prevalent form of payment for people in all income brackets, according to our survey. Obviously, choosing a method of health care is one of the hardest aspects of living in San Miguel for the retirees. According to our survey, 36.5 percent of respondents reported that they have a Mexican source for health care (see Appendix C: Data by Question, Question 2). While others would like to pursue their health care in San Miguel, they return to the U.S. so that Medicare will pay for their medical services. According to our survey, 86.5 percent of respondents in San Miguel reported that they would seek health care in Mexico if Medicare would cover the costs (see Appendix C: Data by Question, Question 13.) Others choose to stay in Mexico for their medical needs, but they must go through the inconvenience or financial strain of paying for new insurance or for the medical services themselves. According to our survey, approximately 85 percent of respondents have not purchased Mexican insurance (see Appendix C: Data by Question, Question 11). Few have bought into the IMSS system of insurance. Many retirees have expressed their desire to claim their Medicare benefits in San Miguel and the surrounding cities of San Luis Potosí and Querétaro, where there are good quality hospitals.

Robert and Betty Shores live in San Miguel de Allende and have written to us regarding their concerns over the inconvenience of not having Medicare coverage in Mexico:

> We just a few days ago signed up for Medicare Part B for the first time. We fear the possibility of something occurring to one (or both) of us that would require long-term attention in the States. This is not to say that we do not have a very good care situation here in San Miguel in the new Hospital de la Fe. They saved my life . . . one night last year. But we were out-of-pocket some US$6,000 (for what I'm sure would have been thirty to fifty thousand dollars in the States).[3]

The Shores also expressed concern over getting to the U.S. in an emergency, commenting that it is just not feasible. While the care in the U.S. that they have encountered is excellent, the $600 to $800 needed to travel to U.S. hospitals is a deterrent to seeking care in the U.S.

Many U.S. citizens in San Miguel have contributed to the Social Security System throughout their lives. They do not understand why they cannot take advantage of their benefits just because they live in Mexico. Extending Medicare coverage to Mexico would grant them the benefits that they paid for and are entitled to, and the coverage in Mexico would cost much less than if these citizens were to travel to the U.S. for care. As one retiree commented on his survey, "I feel we are being ripped off."

Cost of Living

One of the main advantages of living in San Miguel de Allende is the low cost of living compared to the United States. Mexico's per capita income is at best one-sixth of that in the United States.[4] A more conservative estimate of the differences in costs between the two countries is that the cost of living is 25 percent less in Mexico than in the United States.[5] This estimate incorporates equal levels of "comfort"—that is, for U.S. citizens who wish to maintain a relatively similar lifestyle in Mexico to how they lived in the United States, the cost of living is about 25 percent less in Mexico.

The disparity between the two countries is even more evident when seen through each nation's minimum wage laws. In December 1997, the minimum wage in Mexico City was raised to 30.20 pesos per day. At the December 1997 exchange rate of 8.3 pesos to the dollar and an average eight-hour work-day, the wage converts to 45 cents an hour. The minimum wage is even lower in the state of Guanajuato, where San Miguel de Allende is located. This figure contrasts sharply to the minimum wage in the United States of $5.15 an hour in December 1997. The Mexican minimum wage is less than one-tenth of that in the United States.

Looking at housing costs, houses ranging from US$25,000 to nearly $150,000 are available in San Miguel.[6] A larger, relatively comfortable house appears to sell for approximately US$80,000 to $100,000. While housing costs in San Miguel are relatively expensive for the whole of Mexico, they are still comparatively less expensive than in the United States. This difference is more obvious in rental properties. A moderately sized house in San Miguel could rent for approximately US$200 to $250 per month. This price is much lower than housing rents in much of the United States.

Health Care System

Residents of San Miguel, and more specifically, U.S. citizens, can choose from several clinics, hospitals, and independent doctors' offices to seek health services in San Miguel and in surrounding cities. However, choosing a doctor can be especially difficult for U.S. retirees in that the majority of them must deal with cultural and linguistic barriers. In addition, many are suspicious of the quality of Mexican health care. For these reasons, word of mouth is essential for the American community in deciding where to pursue health services. As a result, we have narrowed our investigation to the main hospitals which U.S. citizens in San Miguel have been reported to trust and patronize.

Hospitals In and Around San Miguel

Hospital de la Fe

For those Americans living in San Miguel who choose the Mexican health care system for their needs, there are several options of hospitals open to them. The closest option is the Hospital de la Fe in San Miguel. The hospital opened in 1995 with the financial and administrative support of the American community, and currently some Americans hold positions on the Board of Directors. The hospital is for-profit, although there is a foundation, or *patronato,* that collects funds for the benefit of the hospital. The hospital has 15 beds and usually has at least one patient in residence. While the number of Americans who stay in the hospital are few, many take advantage of the outpatient services. Daily room charges range from $15 for the communal room to $55 for a private room, and the hospital has 22 affiliated physicians.

Hospital de la Fe has a limited supply of medical equipment. They do, however, have X-ray, ultrasound, and dialysis equipment among their supplies. Since the hospital is so small, it is difficult for them to purchase and maintain very sophisticated equipment. They do have basic materials and appear to be equipped to stabilize and transport patients to better-equipped hospitals if necessary.

A current disadvantage of Hospital de la Fe is that cash or credit card are the only forms of payment accepted. The hospital does not accept any type of insurance. This is a factor why many in the American community prefer to pursue their health care in hospitals in surrounding cities.

Hospital San José

Another option for residents of San Miguel is Hospital San José in Querétaro, about 40 miles from San Miguel. With the relatively close proximity and a reputation for high-quality care, this hospital is a favorite option for many San Miguel residents. Hospital San José was founded in 1994 and is owned and operated by the García Borbolla family. The hospital has complete and updated equipment to provide a wide variety of services. It is a fairly large hospital, with 64 beds and a staff of 101 physicians, several of whom have received training in the United States.

The hospital is for-profit. However, there is a non-profit foundation, called *Patronato Médico de San Miguel y San José* that is affiliated with the hospital. The foundation assists people who need medical attention and do not have the money to cover their expenses. This *patronato* has a different function than the one serving the Hospital de la Fe. The *patronato* serving Hospital de la Fe raises funds for the hospital, whereas the one serving Hospital San José raises funds for patients.

Another advantage of Hospital San José is that it has academic exchange agreements with Hermann Hospital in Houston and Methodist Hospital in San Antonio. The hospital hosts visiting physicians from these affiliated hospitals, who give medical presentations.

Fortunately, Hospital San José accepts almost any type of insurance, including both Mexican and American. Among the most common insurance plans accepted are those from *Seguros Monterrey Aetna* and *Seguros Comercial.* In addition, the hospital offers its own insurance plan, called *Protecmédica,* in which people can buy insurance that only covers treatment at Hospital San José.

Due to the high demand for medical services in San Miguel, Hospital San José opened an emergency care unit in San Miguel in November 1997. This unit has an ambulance and medical staff available 24 hours a day. Patients in serious condition are usually stabilized in the emergency unit and then transported to Hospital San José. This service appears to be a welcome addition in San Miguel. Residents have expressed relief that there is an experienced team waiting to transport them to a hospital where their insurance will be accepted.

While many Americans in San Miguel claim to visit and trust the services of Hospital San José, the hospital itself does not record the number of American citizens that it treats. Therefore, it is hard to estimate the actual number of Americans treated at the hospital each year.

Hospital de Nuestra Señora de la Salud

While few Americans from San Miguel currently seek medical care from the Hospital de Nuestra Señora de la Salud in the city of San Luis Potosí, the hospital is worth considering in a project to extend Medicare due to its excellent quality of care. The hospital was established in 1991 and is today considered one of the best in central Mexico. The hospital has established an academic exchange agreement with St. Luke's Episcopal Hospital in Houston and is a participating member of the International Health Care Alliance and of the Texas Heart Institute.

Currently, the hospital has 100 beds and it is expanding to 150 beds. The hospital has 79 affiliated physicians. Daily room charges range from $55 for a double room to $105 for a premium suite. In addition, the hospital accepts several types of insurance, including American insurance plans. While not many Americans visit this hospital, it does have a heliport that would be beneficial in transporting patients to the hospital in emergencies.

This hospital is also for-profit. Approximately 100 stockholders, many of whom are doctors, own the hospital. There are also several *patronatos* that are affiliated with the hospital. These *patronatos* assist people who cannot cover their medical expenses; for example, they may assist people who need organ transplants or other very costly procedures.

Hospital Nuestra Señora de la Salud has many advanced facilities, including a reproductive medicine unit that is one of only three in Mexico. While this unit is not a concern of this project, it is important in evaluating the overall quality of the hospital. In addition, the hospital supports a clinical and a pathology laboratory and it houses several pieces of advanced medical equipment. (Although the imaging equipment is owned by the imaging company that provides the services at the hospital, Mexican physicians often own their own equipment, depending on their specialty.)

The hospital has several features which make it worthy of inclusion in this project. First, the hospital has a heliport that could facilitate transporting U.S. citizens from San Miguel to the hospital, and to the United States if necessary. Second, the hospital frequently uses a large auditorium for talks from visiting physicians from within Mexico and beyond. Therefore, the hospital already has demonstrated great interest in sharing information and establishing links abroad. And third, the hospital estimates that 50 percent of the doctors working with the hospital have studied outside Mexico.[7] While this figure does not indicate degrees earned abroad, it does illustrate that many doctors have a working knowledge of English and the American health care system.

Centro Médico del Potosí

Centro Médico, a nonprofit organization in San Luis Potosí, is another favorite hospital of the American residents of San Miguel de Allende. The hospital, which was established in 1973, is owned by a group of several partners, called an "Anonymous Society." Centro Médico is reputed to employ many of the finest doctors in Mexico. The hospital has 67 beds and 206 affiliated physicians, the most physicians of the four hospitals examined. Daily room charges range from $62 for a shared room to $117.50 for a suite. In addition, the hospital charges the patient approximately $37.50 per day in hospital fees.[8]

Centro Médico appears to have the most advanced equipment on average of all of the hospitals we contacted. The "Anonymous Society" owns all of the equipment used in the hospital. Among other resources, the hospital has several laboratories, including clinical, pathology, bacteriology, hematology, and immunization. In addition, hospital treatments include chemotherapy, radiotherapy, dialysis, laser ophthamology, nuclear medicine, and physical therapy.

The main advantage of Centro Médico for U.S. citizens living in San Miguel is the insurance plan the hospital offers. The plan is offered for either six months or a year. For an individual born between 1923 and 1927, the initial enrollment fee for the year is $1,260. For a person born between 1918 and 1922, the fee is $1,470, and for a person born before 1917, the fee is $1,680. The renewal fee, however, is much lower, at $840 per year, regardless of age. The fees for a married couple are slightly less per person.

Almost everything is covered during a hospital stay, including an individual room, medicines prescribed during the hospital stay, laboratory work, medical and surgery fees, physician fees, nursing care, meals, operating and recovery room, supplies, oxygen, intensive care unit, and transfusions. The enrollee must, however, stay at least one night in the hospital to be covered for most services. In addition, the patient must pay a deductible of $150 each time he or she is committed to the hospital. The enrollee is not covered for fees exceeding $9,375. If fees do exceed this amount, then the patient will receive discounts on the remaining uncovered bills. The hospital comments that on average, less than one person per year has exceeded the maximum allowance. This statistic is important in that it gives an idea of the total costs per patient in Mexico for U.S. retirees.

The enrollee is entitled to certain privileges throughout the year that are not related to hospitalization. The enrollee is allowed free consultations whether or not the consultation results in hospitalization. However, procedures performed during these consultations on an outpatient basis are not covered. Another benefit is if the enrollee has not been hospitalized during the year, then her or she is entitled to a free check-up with an assigned doctor in January of the following year. The check-up includes several tests, including a blood test, urinanalysis, electrocardiogram, chest X-ray, mammogram, prostate exam, and blood pressure test.

While this plan has attracted many residents of San Miguel, it contains many gaps. The plan does not cover stays relating to drug or alcohol abuse, psychiatric care, suicide attempts, malignant blood conditions, chemotherapy, organ transplants, rehabilitation, radiotherapy, or prosthetic, mechanical, or electrical devices. In addition, while other pre-existing conditions are covered through the plan, prostate gland treatment is excluded from coverage during the first year of enrollment. Ambulance fees are also excluded. Many of these exclusions may be vital to retirees. The gaps in coverage could force them to return to the United States for care.

Other Hospitals and Medical Clinics in San Miguel

The San Miguel area has nine additional hospitals and clinics, three of which are available to U.S. retirees and are briefly described below. We have not looked more in depth at these clinics due to the fact that they are not used much by the American population. The remaining clinics are not useful for this study because they are exclusively for indigent youths, government employees (ISSSTE), childbearing women, or have less than eight physicians.

Hospital General is owned by the government of Guanajuato and has 17 physicians. It averages 40 patients per day and accepts cash only. It uses a manual recordkeeping system and is regulated by the Secretaría de Salud. The IMSS hospital is owned and regulated by the federal IMSS system and accepts IMSS insurance only. It employs 12 physicians and averages about 60 patients per day. Sanatorio Torres de San Miguel is owned by Dr. Jose Luís Torres and employs 12 physicians. It averages 16 patients per day and accepts cash only. It also relies on manual recordkeeping and is regulated by the Secretaría de Salud.

Hospital Charges for Several Procedures
The Hospital de la Fe in San Miguel de Allende, the Hospital de Nuestra Señora de la Salud in San Luis Potosí, and Centro Médico in San Luis Potosí have printed price lists for several surgical procedures. These lists include only the hospital fees; there are additional fees for laboratory services, surgeons, anesthesiology, and primary care. For example, Table 4.1 lists the price of an appendectomy at the Hospital de la Fe as $350. The additional fees could total approximately $1,000,[9] bringing the total cost of the procedure to $1,350 plus tax. As one can see, these costs, together with physicians' fees and hospital fees, total only a fraction of the cost of these same procedures in the United States.

Physicians and Nurses

Specialties of Physicians and Nurses
The Hospital de la Fe in San Miguel de Allende has 22 affiliated physicians practicing 20 different specialties. The only specialties with more than one practitioner are cardiology and urology. The hospital also employs 22 nurses, all of whom have received their certification either through the *Universidad Nacional Autónoma de México* (UNAM) or through the nursing schools affiliated with the UNAM or a State Secretariat of Public Education. The closest nursing school to San Miguel is in Celaya. In addition, the hospital runs a

	Table 4.1		
	Comparison of Costs at Three Hospitals (in US $)		
Procedure	Hospital de la Fe	Hospital de Nuestra Señora	Centro Médico del Potosí
Appendectomy	$350	$296	$300
Hernia surgery	250	308	300
Prostate surgery	350	473	450
Tonsillectomy	275	186	212
Laparotomy	412	408	462

Source: Printed price lists from Hospital de la Fe and Hospital de Nuestra Señora, San Miguel de Allende, Mexico, and Centro Médico del Potosí, San Luis Potosí, Mexico, obtained from visits to the hospitals by Horacio Aldrete and Amy Sprague, November 1997.

training program for nurses' aides employed by the hospital. This program lasts two years and is only for those nurses' aides at the Hospital de la Fe.[10]

Centro Médico in San Luis Potosí employs 206 physicians practicing 31 specialties. The specialties with the most practitioners are gynecology (27), pediatrics (23), general surgery (20), and cardiology (16). The hospital nursing staff are categorized into three levels (the exact number of nurses was not available, and the hospital indicated there was a high turnover rate for nurses). The highest level of nurses are the registered nurses who have to be certified by the *Registro Nacional de Profesiones* (National Registry of Professions), a part of the Ministry of Public Education. This certification is called the *Cédula Profesional.* The next category is the general nurses who also have to be certified in nursing by the National Registry of Professions after completing a college nursing degree. The third level is the nurses' helpers, who only need a diploma from a nursing school.[11]

The Hospital de Nùestra Señora de la Salud has 79 physicians practicing 25 specialties. The most popular specialties are cardiology, general surgery, and pediatrics, with seven physicians each, and anesthesiology, gynecology, and neurosurgery, with six physicians each. The hospital employs 70 nurses in four different categories. Similar to Centro Médico, the hospital employs registered nurses and nurses' helpers. In addition, general nurses are divided into two categories: those with a college degree and those without. The general nurses without college training often receive their diplomas from the Red Cross or a community college.[12]

Hospital San José employs 101 physicians in 22 specialties. All of the specialties have five or fewer practitioners each except for gynecology (17), pediatrics (15), and general surgery and trauma (8 each). The hospital employs 63 nurses: 15 work exclusively in the surgery rooms, and 48 work in the hospital as a whole. These nurses include the general nurses and the nurses' helpers described above. The nurses' helpers at the Hospital San José usually receive their degrees from the Red Cross or another independent institution.[13]

Physician Fees and Caseloads

Determining a specific average charge for services provided by physicians in the San Miguel de Allende area is complicated. The lack of a governing body or association that keeps track of this kind of data makes the physicians themselves our only source of information. Furthermore, there is no regulation to set price ceilings for health services provided, so physicians are free to determine their charges based on their own criteria. However, it is important to mention that this condition only prevails in private medical practice. Public health institutions and their personnel work under a system of fixed pricing where physicians have a preset charge for each type of procedure.

The data used to determine the average charges for care are based solely on the information provided by some of the physicians in the cities of San Miguel de Allende, San Luis Potosí, and Querétaro. At the Hospital de la Fe, the physicians charge an average of US$22 to $25 for a consultation. The patient pays the physician directly for his or her services. Each physician sees an average of ten to fifteen patients daily, three to four of whom are U.S. citizens.

We received estimates for consultation charges from three doctors in San Luis Potosí: Dr. Jorge Rodríguez Barrios, subdirector of the Hospital de Nuestra Señora; Dr. Pedro Rosales Pérez, a pediatrician; and Dr. Antonio Cano Gómez, a general practitioner in San Luis Potosí. They estimate that a general practitioner charges approximately $15 per visit, a pediatrician charges approximately $25 per visit, and other specialists charge approximately $35 per visit. These charges are relatively the same as those in San Luis Potosí. Physicians at Centro Médico del Potosí charge an average of $25 per visit. This fee appears to be relatively constant throughout the specialties.[14]

Nursing Homes

In San Miguel, there are only a few nursing homes. However, the American population does not utilize these facilities because they are exclusively for the indigent elderly of San Miguel. They have been built to provide only basic services. The Hospital de la Fe has developed plans to build a nursing home as an addition to the hospital that would also provide hospice care and that would be open to both the American and Mexican residents of San Miguel. The plans are currently on hold due to a lack of funds.

It is hard to estimate the demand for the nursing home, but according to Dr. Arturo Barrera at the Hospital de la Fe, there are several elderly Americans and Mexicans who live alone "who should not have to do so."[15] However, according to Jim Austin, the owner of MediPlan in Guadalajara, a typical American in Mexico who needs to move into a nursing home would prefer to return to the United States to receive this care rather than stay in Mexico at a lower cost.[16]

Home Health

An informal home health care system is available to residents of San Miguel, but the majority of these home health care workers are not trained in the health professions.[17] Furthermore, there are no agencies that regulate home health care, and workers are found and hired through word of mouth and personal recommendations. This is an informal system in which there are plenty of people looking for these in-home employment opportunities. The price of an in-home helper is approximately US$40 per week. For those who need limited extra help in their homes, San Miguel provides this cheap alternative to home health.

Pharmacies and Medications

With 34 pharmacies in San Miguel de Allende, 64 in Querétaro, and 248 in San Luis Potosí, the pharmacy business remains competitive.[18] Many are very small pharmacies (*boticas*) that on the whole only accept cash. However, the larger pharmacies accept both cash and credit cards, and the ISSSTE pharmacies accept special government coupons as payment. Following is a comparison of the prices of several commonly prescribed drugs in the United States and in San Luis Potosí. These prices are generally similar to those in the other areas studied in Mexico. Most pharmaceuticals in Mexico are cheaper than their counterparts in the U.S., but there are a few which for various reasons are more expensive.

Table 4.2
Sample Pharmaceutical Prices in Mexico and the U.S.

Drug Name (name in Mexico if different)	Purpose	San Luis Potosí (converted to US$)	United States
Augmentin: 500 mg, 15 tabs	antibiotic	$21.68	$55.51
Axid: 150 mg, 60 tabs	treat ulcers	29.59	84.21
Capoten (Capotena): 25 mg, 100 tabs	treat high blood pressure	40.62	69.27
Ceclor: 250 mg, 30 tabs	antibiotic	26.39	57.84
Pepcid (Pepcidine): 20 mg, 60 tabs	treat ulcers	36.09	84.12
Premarin: 0.625 mg, 100 tabs	hormone replacement	39.32	40.94
Prozac: 20 mg, 100 tabs	treat depression	32.58	201.09
Tagamet: 300 or 400 mg,* 60 tabs	treat ulcers	13.95	54.15
Zovirax: 200 mg, 100 tabs	treat herpes virus	126.78	94.88

Sources: Mexican prices obtained by Rafael Manuel Aldrete Coronado from Botica Mexico and Farmacia ISSSTE in San Luis Potosí, Mexico, April 1998 (prices given are the average of the two pharmacies); U.S. prices from Internet Discount Pharmacy, "U-Save Pharmacy Product Price Examples," http://www.capc.com/usave/specials.cgi. Accessed: February 2, 1998.

* Price based on 400 mg strength in Mexican pharmacies and 300 mg strength in U.S. pharmacies.

Notes

1. Telephone interview by Amy Sprague with Philip Maher, United States Consular Agent, San Miguel de Allende, Mexico, October 3, 1997.

2. LBJ School Survey of U.S. Retirees in Mexico, San Miguel de Allende, 1998.

3. Robert and Betty Shores, "Medicare Coverage," Personal email to Horacio Aldrete, April 6, 1998.

4. Christopher Reynolds, "Annual Tours for the Thinking Person: Latin America; Off to Learn the Lingo; In Mexico and Latin America, How to Choose the Best Place to Learn Spanish," *Los Angeles Times* (January 11, 1998), p. L1.

5. Jack Anderson, "Many American Retirees" (editorial), *The State Journal-Register* (Springfield, Ill., August 23, 1996), p. 10.

6. Classified advertisements, *Atención San Miguel,* Real Estate section, November 3, 1997.

7. Interview by Horatio Aldrete and Amy Sprague with Dr. Jorge Rodríguez Barrios, Medical Director, Hospital de Nuestra Señora de la Salud, San Luis Potosí, Mexico, November 8, 1997.

8. Printout of prices supplied by Centro Médico del Potosí, San Luis Potosí, Mexico, November 1997, n.p.

9. Dr. Arturo Barrera, Hospital de la Fe, "Re: Los costas," Personal email to Amy Sprague, April 13, 1998.

10. Ibid., "Re: Doctores y Entermeras," March 11, 1998.

11. Telephone interview by Horacio Aldrete with Licenciado Miguel Angel Carranco, Director General, Centro Médico del Potosí, San Luis Potosí, Mexico, April 16, 1998.

12. Rodríguez interview.

13. Telephone interview by Horatio Aldrete with Enrique Borbolla, General Director, Hospital San José, April 7, 1998.

14. Printout of prices supplied by Centro Médico del Potosí.

15. Dr. Arturo Barrera, Hospital de la Fe, "Nursing Homes," Personal email to Amy Sprague, February 6, 1998.

16. Class presentation by Jim Austin, owner of MediPlan, Denver, Colorado, at the Lyndon B. Johnson School of Public Affairs, Austin, Texas, February 9, 1998.

17. Telephone interview by Amy Sprague with Roger Allen, head of the American Legion, San Miguel de Allende, Mexico, February 4, 1998.

18. Telephone directories for the cities of San Miguel de Allende, Querétaro, and San Luis Potosí, Mexico, 1994.

Chapter 5
Guadalajara and the Lake Chapala Area

by Olga Oralia Garcia and Lauren Lacefield Lewis

A MERICANS WHO LIVE OUTSIDE THE UNITED STATES IN GUADALAJARA AND the Lake Chapala area are fortunate to live inexpensively in beautiful cities with a wide variety of services available to meet their social and health needs. Since Guadalajara is the second-largest city in Mexico, it has several hospitals, many clinics, and a large number of independent physicians and nurses. The people of Mexico enjoy low-cost health care provided by professionals who often spend extra time with their patients and still make house calls. This fact, coupled with their preference for in-home as opposed to long-term institutional care for the elderly, has shaped the infrastructure of health care in this region. Many Americans who have retired in the Guadalajara area are in a position to take advantage of excellent lifestyles and good health care at greatly reduced prices. Furthermore, the United States government has the opportunity to provide a substantial benefit to its citizens by allowing them freedom of movement, freedom of choice, and decreased cost for medical care.

Although it is not known how many foreigners have retired to Mexico, clearly there are large numbers of Americans residing in this region. If the Lake Chapala Society, whose membership is largely American, can attract 1,600 members[1] and the American Society in Guadalajara could attract 3,000 members[2] at its peak, there must be a substantial community of Americans whose lives would be greatly improved by having the option to use their Medicare benefits in Mexico.

Unofficial Estimates of the Retired American Population

One of the most difficult questions addressed by our project has been determining a good estimate of the number of Medicare-eligible persons residing in Mexico. This question is difficult to answer for several reasons: many persons reside in Mexico permanently yet do not obtain visas indicating permanent residency, most eligible retirees have their social security checks delivered within U.S. borders, and many fail to register at the American Embassy.[3] The problem is exacerbated by the large number of Canadians who have settled in this region (who may be mistaken for Americans) and the large number of visiting Americans who spend the winter months in this area each year.

There are conflicting estimates of the number of retired Americans living in this region. For example, the American Embassy in Guadalajara estimates that there are 50,000 Americans living in the Guadalajara and Lake Chapala area.[4] In contrast, the local English-language newspaper, the *Guadalajara Colony Reporter,* estimates that the American population is only 15,000 overall, with 8,000 over 65 years of age.[5] The *Colony Reporter* bases its estimates on figures provided by Javier Dueñas, the director of the Immigration Department. In an interview, Sr. Dueñas indicated that only 13,000 Americans residing in the Guadalajara area have residency papers. It was also estimated that 7,000 of these Americans are younger than retirement age.[6]

Population

Do you ever wonder what happened to your first-grade teacher, or where your mailman is now that he has retired? These days you can find everyday people like these living alongside people who fought in World War II and those who have explored the globe their entire lives. When we sat down to talk to Americans living in Guadalajara and the Lake Chapala area, we heard stories of wives who were cryptographers in WWII, women who piloted small aircraft, and couples who had spent 50 years raising a family together.

According to the 1997-1998 LBJ School Survey of U.S. Retirees in Mexico, the American retirees in the Guadalajara-Lake Chapala area stated that their primary reasons for living in Mexico were cost of living, climate, the culture, and the people as well as the social opportunities (see Appendix C: Data by Question, Question 26). We spoke to many people who plan to stay in Mexico the rest of their lives. They indicate that nothing short of revolution or economic collapse would force them out. The weather is beautiful, the arts and history abound, and almost everyone indicated what a joy it was that you could eat a first-class meal at an excellent restaurant for 60 pesos, which is approximately seven U.S. dollars. "People here walk more, travel more, swim more. The big danger is people eat more because it is so cheap," said one retiree.[7]

Transitions

Americans and Mexicans living in Guadalajara and the Lake Chapala area have constructed an infrastructure that helps support Americans newly arriving in this area. A strong infrastructure is important, since many Americans are settling in this region. Americans can be found in almost every colonia in Guadalajara and in every new development around the Lake Chapala area. Serving this dispersed population, the English-language newspaper the *Guadalajara Colony Reporter* has a circulation between 6,000 and 7,000 in the winter and 5,000 in the summer.[8] In addition, the Lake Chapala area is served by a free monthly magazine called *El Ojo del Lago*. These two papers are widely circulated among retirees in the area and are a good source of news and information.

There are also small networks of small-business people that are often key for helping retirees adapt to their new environment. For example, there is a small grocery store called "David's" in Chapalita, a colonia of Guadalajara, owned by a Canadian man and his Mexican wife. They also own several small apartments that are rented by some Americans, and the wife, Carmen, does hair in a two-chair beauty shop and runs a small flower stall.[9] People really seem to appreciate close-knit relationships such as these.

Groups
It is estimated that there are over 80 English-speaking social, fraternal, religious, special-interest, and charitable groups in the Guadalajara-Lake Chapala area.[10] Five of the largest groups are the American Legion at Lake Chapala and in Guadalajara, the Lake Chapala Society, the American Society in Guadalajara, and the International Friendship Club. The Lake Chapala Society has a membership of over 2,300 and the American Society in Guadalajara has boasted a membership of 3,000 at its highest.

Each of these groups serves different purposes in its community. The International Friendship Club primarily supports the young wives of U.S. executives living in Mexico. The two American Legion groups host large breakfasts, picnics, dances, and many types of game-playing. They are also very involved in fundraising to support local charities. The American Legion has established a health plan where Legion members can use local military hospitals.[11]

The American Society in Guadalajara (AMSOC), founded in 1945, offers everything from Unitarian meetings with outside speakers to Spanish classes, dances, and literary groups. For example, they host "Aloud," which is a group of people who like to read aloud. They read one-act plays, short stories, and poetry while enjoying snacks and wine.[12]

The Lake Chapala Society, founded in 1953, has an amazing array of support services including group medical, home, and car insurance through Aetna; post-life planning; video rentals; free eye exams; and free blood pressure and diabetes screening.[13] In addition, there is a computer club, a ham radio club, and a writers' group as well as exercise and Spanish classes.[14]

Everyday Life in Guadalajara

Many features of everyday life in Guadalajara and Lake Chapala make them feel a little more like home to many Americans. There are places like Sandy's Bookstore, which is well stocked with English language books. Plaza Del Sol is a mall with modern clothing, houseware, and jewelry stores. A favorite hang-out is Sanborn's, which has food much like a Denny's, where many older gentlemen spend a good portion of their mornings together talking over coffee.

Plaza Del Sol has a large combination grocery and department store known as Gigante where, besides shopping, people can pay their telephone and electric bills.[15] For the more traditional, there are abundant local markets and corner stores where shopping is a bit less "Americanized." In addition, Guadalajara showcases world-class theatre and the arts. There is an amazing array of beautiful architecture with great historical significance all over Guadalajara, and there are small squares where families gather in the evenings to listen to local orchestras.

Everyday Life in the Lake Chapala Area

The Chapala-area communities are situated around Lake Chapala, Mexico's largest inland lake. Although Chapala is not a large metropolis, it has four car rental companies, hardware stores, pool supply centers, and nurseries.[16] Many feel that the atmosphere is more relaxed in the Lake Chapala area than in Guadalajara.

Many residents of Chapala do their major shopping once a month in Guadalajara in places such as Gigante or Wal-Mart. Lakeside also has two local grocery stores that have been compared to large convenience stores. There are also small Mexican groceries where you can find eggs, meat, and some canned goods, and a plaza nearby where fresh fruit and vegetables can be purchased.

Shopping in the Lake Chapala area is characterized by flea markets and small artisan shops. There are three golf courses in the Chapala area, a public tennis court in Christiana Park, and the Ajijic Racquet Club. The lakeside Little Theatre in Chula Vista makes English presentations throughout the tourist season.

Publications such as the *Mexico Living and Travel Newsletter* use the economical prices in Guadalajara as a major selling point for moving to Mexico. In the Spring 1997 issue it quoted some average prices as follows (all prices in U.S. dollars):[17]

- Premium gasoline: $1.43 per gallon

- Woman's perm and haircut: $17.18

- Electricity: $12.85 per month

- Propane gas for cooking: $12.59 per month

- Telephone basic service: $9.59 per month

- Water for drinking: $5.50 per month

- Thorough housecleaning (4-5 hours): $6.36 per visit

- Dry cleaning (pants or skirt): $1.72

- Whole chicken: $.95

- Hamburger : $1.73 per pound

- Potatoes: $.36 per pound

- Oranges: $.10 per pound

- Margarine: $1.37

- Flour: $1.01

- Eggs (dozen): $1.13

- 2 liters Coca-Cola: $.85

- 2 liters milk: $.97

- Veterinarian consultation: $10

Many people consider this area to be ideally suited to people living on limited incomes. For example, grocery stores let customers purchase needed items in small quantities, such as buying broccoli or celery by the individual stalk.[18] In addition, Guadalajara boasts an extensive bus system, meaning that retirees do not need to own cars. Buses can take people to local malls, restaurants, and grocery stores for as little as two pesos. Most people in

Guadalajara indicate that they live no more than two blocks from the nearest bus stop.[19]

In addition, we spoke to many people who go dancing every week at the Legion or American Society and women assured us that they felt much safer in Mexico than they had in the United States. We interviewed women who said they feel safe walking their dogs at 10 or 11 o'clock at night.

Income

The people who come to Mexico from the U.S. to retire are not a homogenous group. Twenty percent of the retirees in Guadalajara who responded to our survey reported an annual income of less than $15,000, 35.3 percent reported an annual income between $15,000 and $25,000, 17.6 percent reported an annual income between $25,000 and $35,000, and 22.4 reported an annual income greater than $35,000 (see Appendix C: Data by Question, Question 27). Some are very well off, yet those who are not wealthy seem to live very well and are certainly better off than if they had remained in the United States on their small incomes.

We spoke to one woman who is living on a limited income—she has budgeted only US$600 per month to live on.[20] She indicates that if she does not buy much meat, she usually has some money left over. She spends about US$220 per month on rent and under US$400 on everything else. She is trying to reduce her long-distance telephone bills but still talks on the phone a good amount. In a recent month she spent 459 pesos, about 40 U.S. dollars, on telephone service. She sold her house when she left the U.S. and has enough on her current budget to live four years in Mexico. Her Social Security allowance begins in three and a half years so if she stays on her budget she will be fine. She may live on a small budget but she is having a great time in Mexico. She is enjoying art classes, where she has learned silverworking, glassworking, and painting. She goes dancing often and goes out on dates.

We spoke to another woman who spends about 15,000 pesos per month, less than US$2,000.[21] She had worked consistently as a legal secretary her whole adult life but had never been able to afford her own washer and dryer in the U.S. Now she has a nice two-bedroom apartment in a good neighborhood for 1,600 pesos a month (about 200 U.S. dollars). She lives within walking distance of her good friend's apartment. She enjoys world-class symphonies, piano recitals, opera, and the ballet. She even has a brand-new washer and dryer.

Some people come to Mexico after substantial careers. We spoke to one woman who had been a lobbyist and an assistant to the chief executive of a major foundation.[22] She had saved consistently through her 401(k) savings plan but realized after speaking to a financial advisor that if she retired in 1993 to Washington or Florida her standard of living would decrease significantly. So, she put her house on the market and gave away most of her possessions, then drove to Mexico with her son, clothes, computer, printer, sheets, and towels. She has now bought wonderful furniture from local artisans and has decorated her attractive, medium-sized home with local art. Her home, which rents for 4,200 pesos per month (about 500 U.S. dollars), is built around a small garden atrium. She generally spends only about US$1,000 per month and is considered a middle-income resident.

Like many of the people we spoke to, this retiree stays very busy. She is active on the board of the American Society in Guadalajara, goes to the AMSOC Friday night socials, and plays Skipbo at AMSOC on Thursday afternoons. She is also involved with the American Legion Auxiliary, which does a lot of fundraising for charity. She goes to the American Legion for breakfast on Saturday mornings and attends their picnics. She also goes to the bullfights every Sunday in the late afternoon when they are in season.

There are some who have come to Mexico even though they could live quite well in the United States. We interviewed one couple who moved to Guadalajara as part-time residents.[23] They sold their large house in Washington, D.C., and moved to New York where the wife's grown children live. Their niece is an architect in Puerto Vallarta and they have children in California. In addition, the husband has two sisters who live in Mexico. Living half of the year in Mexico seemed like the perfect way to keep in touch with family members and enjoy a wonderful climate.

This couple indicated that they spend about the same amount of money as they do in the United States but live better in Mexico. They generally spend about $80,000 U.S. dollars per year. Although they could easily afford to purchase a nice house, the couple purchased a three-bedroom condominium seven years ago, paying about US$62,000. They also own the apartment next door, which they currently rent out. In the future, they plan to rent it to someone who will care for them as they age. They live in a gated community of houses and condominiums. They pay 2,500 pesos per month in homeowners' fees for gardening, building repairs, lights, and security. Their neighborhood is filled with luxurious homes that would not be out of place in the nicest exclusive neighborhoods in the United States.

The couple lives near a country club whose members are primarily native Mexicans. Each morning the husband rises early to work out at the club, then enjoys a steam bath and jacuzzi. He eats breakfast with a group of friends and works part-time at the local university. While he goes to Mass Sunday morning his wife eats outside in the garden. He also sings in a choir at the country club while his wife plays bridge. The husband writes poetry and his wife knits sweaters for the indigenous children who live up in the mountains where it is cold.

Unfortunately, life in Mexico becomes more difficult once you can no longer pay your bills independently, require constant medical care, and need someone to check on you.[24] Some people are fortunate and have a good friend who helps make sure that everything is taken care of. But for most, the American Society in Guadalajara has a committee that looks in on the homebound. If these individuals go to poverty hospitals, the American Society sends someone to help them to the bathroom and feed them. They may even provide assistance for those in the larger hospitals where the family instead of nurses is expected to help patients with many of these functions. When a person becomes too incapacitated to live on his or her own, the American Society helps people take care of their business and close their homes in Mexico and return to the United States.[25]

One gentleman tells a story of the days when he was very young and studying in Boston and he did not have enough money to buy an overcoat. Now, he and his wife have assets of over one million dollars and are living very well in Mexico. The people we spoke with had incredible stories to tell about lifetimes of struggles, successes, and hard work. Most are quick to point out that they still pay their U.S. taxes and that they paid their entire lifetime into a health care system that they are unable to utilize while living in Mexico.

American retirees are looking for a place where they can enjoy everything that they have worked to achieve. Many are open about the fact that they wish to die with dignity in a place that is beautiful, where people respect the elderly, and where they are among friends. Unfortunately, it is the lack of support for their health care needs that makes this difficult for many Americans living abroad.

Health Care System

The health care system in Mexico is constantly changing in order to address the needs of all those living within its borders. Some American retirees who responded to our survey in Guadalajara and Chapala had personal perspectives on the health care services available in Mexico. For example, an American physician retired in Mexico commented, "I am a physician impressed with medical care here [Guadalajara] where there is not the threat of medical malpractice suits being held over the heads of physicians. Doctors are humanely oriented first, laboratory second."[26] A couple of survey respondents made comments about IMSS such as "[I am] happy with IMSS, except for long waiting lines"[27] and "IMSS offers a lot for the price."[28] Many American retirees seem comfortable with the Mexican health care system. In fact, our results found that 62.4 percent of the 83 Americans retirees responding to the survey in the Guadalajara area have a Mexican source for health care. Only

28.2 percent have returned to the United States for care (see Appendix C: Data by Questions, Questions 2 and 8).

Mexico is slowly becoming more aware of the health needs of its elderly population. In the year 2030, 15.2 million, or 11.7 percent of the Mexican population, are expected to be 65 years or older.[29] Research in this area will help Mexican health institutions deal with thousands of retired American citizens throughout Mexico as well. A 1993 Mexican study, published by Salud Publica de Mexico (Public Health in Mexico), showed that 79 percent of the elderly who live in urban areas and 67 percent who live in suburban areas used health services within the last 12 months.[30] For elderly men, the average hospital stay was 16.5 days and for females over 60 years old, 14.8 days.[31] The most frequent utilization of hospitals was due to old age chronic illness.[32] Even though this study examined all the elderly people who utilized health services in Mexico, it may be an indicator that American retirees who live in the urban areas are also strong users of a variety of medical services, especially in a city full of medical services such as Guadalajara. According to the Mexican National Health Survey II, only an estimated 2.4 percent of the elderly Mexican population have private Mexican insurance.[33] Many American retirees tend to rely on either a pension fund or Social Security or both. Many Americans are not able to buy private health insurance if they only have modest pension or Social Security benefits. Therefore, the percentage of American retirees with private health insurance may be similar to that of Mexican nationals holding private health insurance. Socioeconomic factors have a great deal to do with the health status of the elderly population in Mexico. The greater the resources available to the Mexican elderly, the better health they are able to maintain.[34] This might also hold true for the different socioeconomic classes of American retirees in Mexico.

Hospitals

According to the 1993 National Census of Private Hospitals in Mexico, of 2,723 total private hospitals in Mexico, only 101 had 30 to 49 hospital beds and only 90 private hospitals had over 50 beds. Ninety-three percent of the private hospitals had 29 beds or fewer.[35] However, private hospitals have more beds overall than other medical clinics or public hospitals. In this 1993 study, private hospitals had 33,397 beds, IMSS had 28,142 beds, SSA had 22,882 beds, ISSSTE had 6,160 beds, the government had 6,730 beds, and other entities, such as clinics, had 8,769 beds.[36] Also according to the 1993 hospital census, Jalisco State had 2,822 private hospital beds in 137 private hospitalization units and 59.1 percent of them had fewer than 15 beds.[37] A number of private hospitals in Guadalajara have succeeded in maintaining high standards for both their own population and the thousands of American retirees in the area. According to a survey respondent,

"[Patients receive] excellent care in medical facilities. You are treated as a patient here with warmth."[38]

According to Geraldine Cortez, the Federal Benefits Director at the American Consulate in Guadalajara, Americans in the greater Guadalajara area tend to frequent three main hospitals: Hospital Mexico-Americano, Hospital Del Carmen, and Hospital Sharp Americas. In addition, Hospital San Javier, constructed three years ago, has also become an option for wealthier American retirees wishing to use its advanced technology.

The following is a brief description of the aforementioned hospitals. The information covered will include ownership and/or affiliations, total bed count, average census, average number of American patients, daily room charges, types of payment accepted, standard recordkeeping practices, and American hospitals that have established working relationships with the respective Mexican hospitals.

Hospital Mexico-Americano

Hospital Mexico-Americano was started by a group of American physicians about 40 years ago.[39] Originally, only U.S. physicians worked at the hospital. Eventually, many Mexican physicians became attracted to Hospital Mexico-Americano because of the opportunities for learning American medicine from the U.S. physicians. Mexican physicians now constitute the majority at the hospital. Many of the original clientele were of U.S. origin and were attracted to the hospital for several reasons. The original staff of physicians was trained in the United States, spoke English, and understood different billing methods, such as CHAMPUS (now Tricare). The hospital staff's familiarity with veterans' benefits was especially helpful for the Vietnam War veterans retiring in Guadalajara in the 1970s. The hospital's clientele has shifted since then in that though American retirees still utilize this hospital, the majority of the patients are of Mexican origin.[40]

Hospital Mexico-Americano treats about 5,000 patients a year.[41] The average number of American retirees treated each year is difficult to estimate because Americans fall into one or more of the categories below:

- locals with private health insurance;

- Americans with a pension;

- American veterans; and

- *particulares,* which is the Spanish term for locals who pay with cash and who tend to blend in with the Mexican population, regardless of their ethnic background.

The hospital has a total of 80 usable beds and the daily room charges vary. Hospital Mexico-Americano accepts many forms of payment. The most common insurance used by American retirees is Tricare and Blue Cross/Blue Shield drawn from throughout the United States. ChampVA, the program that covers veterans with a service-connected disability anywhere in the world for services related to that disability, is also used. According to the September 1997 Tricare Standard Handbook, administration of ChampVA is the sole responsibility of the Veterans Health Administration Center in Denver, Colorado.[42] This includes the determination of eligibility, the authorization of benefits, and the processing of claims. According to Esperanza Herrera, who has been the billing officer at Mexico-Americano for over 25 years, all U.S. veterans need authorization from the Denver office before relocating in order to receive health benefits abroad. United States federal employees working at the American Consulate in Guadalajara also have their own insurance, American Services, which is billed directly by the hospital for any medical services. In general, cash, credit card, and/or private Mexican insurance companies are more widely utilized to pay for medical services.[43]

All patients must pay every third day for services rendered at Hospital Mexico-Americano.[44] Neither monthly payments nor any other type of payment plan is available. Different billing procedures are followed for each company, since each patient usually has different insurance contracts that only cover specific medical procedures. All Blue Cross/Blue Shield insurance is accepted from the United States as long as a three-digit authorization code is on the insurance card. This authorization code allows Hospital Mexico-Americano to bill directly. Authorization usually occurs within two to three days. CHAMPUS and other veterans' benefits are billed directly through the CHAMPUS office located in Denver, Colorado, as described above. Tricare, which is the coverage received by military dependents and veterans before they are eligible for Medicare, is billed through Wisconsin Physicians Service.[45] All patient records are kept for five years after the patient's last hospital visit.

According to Dr. Omar Aguilar, Hospital Mexico-Americano has maintained close working relationships with many Baptist-affiliated American hospitals in Texas such as Baylor Hospital in Dallas, Baptist Health System in San Antonio, Hendricks Hospital in Abilene, Methodist Hospital in Houston, Valley Baptist Hospital in Harlingen, and Hillcrest Hospital in Waco.[46] Physicians at Hospital Mexico-Americano and the aforementioned hospitals in the United States help each other with skill development through professional interchanges, holding conferences and workshops both in the United States and Mexico.[47]

Hospital Del Carmen

Hospital Del Carmen was started in 1949 as a maternity hospital and had a religious affiliation.[48] According to Dr. Jaime Ramírez Parra, the chair of the

Division of Gastroenterology, Hospital Del Carmen is the "oldest, but always advancing its technology." It has gradually expanded and is now a hospital offering many different medical services. The physicians who have become members of Hospital Del Carmen are themselves owners of the hospital because they each own a share of the hospital stock.[49] According to Dr. Ramírez, most doctors at Hospital Del Carmen are graduates of Autonoma in Guadalajara and 80 percent have a postgraduate degree either from a major university in Mexico or the United States. He believes the experience of the physicians at Del Carmen is exceptional and far beyond any other hospital in Guadalajara. A credentials committee at Hospital Del Carmen reviews the application of any physician who wants to be on staff. An 80-percent consensus of the committee is needed for approval. All doctors also routinely go through a peer review process, and group diagnostic exercises are common.[50] The nursing staff is also exceptional; according to Dr. Javier Michel Ochoa, the Medical Director at Hospital Del Carmen, the hospital's "biggest asset is the nurses."[51]

Hospital Del Carmen treats an average of 1,000 to 1,500 patients a year, which is over 120 patients a month. The hospital checks in about four Americans per month.[52] A total of 86 beds are located in the hospital (110 total if surgery and infant beds are included). The cost for a room ranges from N$447 to over N$990 a day depending on the comfort level desired by the patient and how many extras are included (such as a private room, additional decoration, privately controlled air conditioning, a private television, and a guest lobby outside the patient's room).[53]

Cash and credit card are the most common forms of payment at Hospital Del Carmen.[54] The hospital has recently begun to accept Blue Cross/Blue Shield of Texas and other U.S. states. (Texas Blue Cross/Blue Shield is currently setting up an international office to help with international billing procedures; Blue Cross/Blue Shield offices in other states are beginning to organize their international billing in a similar manner.) Before any service is provided to a patient at the hospital, a deposit is required. The amount of the deposit depends on the cost of the medical procedure: the more expensive the service, the higher the deposit required prior to any medical services being rendered. After medical services are performed, the balance is required to be paid in full. If the patient is going to be in the hospital for additional days, the hospital bill has to be paid at the end of each week. All patient records are kept for five years after the patient's last hospital visit.[55]

Hospital San Javier

Hospital San Javier is owned by Grupo Empresarial San Javier, which also owns medical equipment, ambulance services, and pharmacies.[56] In addition, Grupo Empresarial San Javier has arrangements with physician groups and other medical-related companies. They pride themselves in having some of the best-trained doctors in Guadalajara. The hospital staff consists of 125 physicians. In addition, 200 other medical associates are allowed to see patients at Hospital San Javier. All physicians are required to have more than just their license and specialty. According to Dr. Carlos Rodríguez Zárate, advanced degrees and additional medical training are required in order to become part of the hospital staff. Hospital San Javier is one of the newest and most technologically advanced hospitals in all of Mexico. It wants to offer the best technology and medical equipment, especially for patients who do not want to go all the way to the United States for medical treatment. American retirees from as far away as Puerto Vallarta request the services at Hospital San Javier due to its medical equipment.[57]

Hospital San Javier is currently filled to capacity and has a waiting list. In 1997 about 6,500 patients were treated. The high occupancy rate is expected to continue as more people hear about the well-trained staff of physicians and the high-quality medical equipment available. The average number of Americans treated each year is about 20 patients. Some of these 20 are American retirees who are willing and able to pay the high costs associated with the hospital.[58]

Hospital San Javier owns 56 regular beds and 88 specialty operating beds. The range in prices is quite wide. Junior rooms run at US$100 a day. These rooms consist of a television, another bed for the spouse or family member, and a complete bathroom. The hospital also has seven master rooms that cost US$1,500 a day. The master bedroom has a spacious waiting area in addition to the items mentioned in the junior rooms, and the large price difference is mostly due to this waiting area.[59]

Cash and credit cards are the most common types of payment accepted at Hospital San Javier. Private Mexican national insurance is accepted as well as international insurance, such as Blue Cross/Blue Shield from different American states. Since the contract with Blue Cross/Blue Shield is relatively recent, the hospital is taking extra precautions in order to ensure payment. Both the authorization and payment periods have proved to take extremely long, and the billing difficulties tend to make Hospital San Javier a bit hesitant about accepting some international insurance coverage. Each patient record contains information about interconsulting among physicians, basic patient medical history, basic patient vital signs, and all services given to the patient.[60]

Hospital San Javier has working relationships with Methodist Hospital in San Antonio, Texas, with St. Joseph in Phoenix, Arizona, and the Mayo Clinic in Rochester, Minnesota.[61] According to Frances Ortiz Schultschik of the Methodist Health Care Systems, Methodist Hospital in San Antonio has created a particularly effective partnership with Hospital San Javier.[62] For example, staff doctors from San Javier Hospital are admitted into the visiting physician program for a period of two weeks to two months. Hospital San

Javier pays for the transportation costs of its staff physician and Methodist Hospital provides room and board at the hospital. Mexican physicians learn new techniques from American physicians doing their rounds, and a panel of physicians at Methodist Hospital works with the visiting physician program to develop more efficient training for the Mexican doctors while in the United States. Even though Mexican physicians do not treat patients in the United States, they assist the American physicians with diagnosing the patient. In addition to the physician education program, staff nurses from Hospital San Javier are also invited to Methodist Hospital for intensive training programs.[63]

Hospital Sharp Americas

Hospital Sharp Americas is affiliated with the Sharp hospital systems in California.[64] An average of 20 to 30 patients are treated each month. A large percentage of its patient base is American retirees. The bed count at Hospital Sharp Americas is ten. The daily room charges are negotiable, and the most common form of payment is through Medicare supplements. According to Dr. Moisés Hernández Nuno, the process of actually receiving payment takes anywhere from six to twelve months. As a result, the hospital charges higher fees than other private hospitals in the area. Because of the smaller number of beds at Hospital Sharp Americas, it might be considered more of a clinic than a hospital.[65]

Mexican Physicians

Many doctors practicing medicine in Mexican private hospitals have specialties in pediatrics, general surgery, gynecology-obstetrics, and internal medicine.[66] Most private hospitals in Mexico tend to have at least a few specialists in each medical field. In 1990 there were a total of 12,457 physicians in the state of Jalisco.[67] It is very rare for a physician not to have a specialty in Guadalajara, especially since "Mexico is saturated with doctors."[68] According to Dr. Ramírez, there is one doctor for every 100 to 150 people in Guadalajara. General practitioners are becoming increasingly rare. Physicians who wish to practice in any Mexican hospital must be the Mexican equivalent to United States board-certified as well. Many promotions in the medical field were once granted on the basis of social class, but though some of these practices may still occur, the majority of the physicians in the best hospitals in Guadalajara are promoted on the basis of merit, continued education, and contributions to the medical field.[69]

Most of the top private hospitals require that physicians practicing in their respective areas come in with strong credentials. For example, Hospital Del Carmen has two different ways of admitting physicians into its staff.[70] Distinguished and reputable physicians may be invited to become part of the staff, while less experienced doctors may buy stock in the hospital after applying and being admitted by a committee of staff physicians. The authorization committee requires an academic curriculum be provided, proof of a medical degree from an accredited medical school, several years of extensive training in a specialty, and a review of the candidate's professional ethics.[71] The authorization committee, under the leadership of Dr. Javier Ochoa, reviews the applications and makes a decision whether to accept a physician or not. Professional ethics and medical experience are the main decision factors.[72] In addition to many of the requirements discussed above, Hospital Mexico-Americano tends to look highly upon a physician having a specialty or experience practicing medicine in the United States. As a result, 50 percent of the active physicians at Hospital Mexico-Americano speak English.[73] The Committee of Credentials at Hospital San Javier actively seeks physicians who have studied in another country, participated in postgraduate work, displayed depth and breadth in their medical education, and have research experience. English-language proficiency is also a plus. Currently, 75 percent of the physicians at San Javier have a working knowledge of English.[74]

Most physicians are involved in informal group practices for the convenience of sharing rent and the salary and services of a secretary. Other physicians find partners in order to jointly buy expensive medical equipment.[75] However, formal contracts between different physician groups usually do not exist. The concepts of preferred provider organizations (PPOs) or health maintenance organizations (HMOs) are not as common in Mexico as they have become in the United States.[76] Even though an American-owned HMO, known as MediPlan, was recently created in Guadalajara, the general idea of HMOs continues to be a novelty. The types of relationships found in American PPOs, however, are beginning to develop. For example, Dr. Compoy from Hospital San Javier, Dr. Ramírez from Hospital Del Carmen, and Dr. Zambrano have each established working relationships with a distinct group of doctors very similar to the practice in a PPO. Dr. Compoy works with a group of 15 physicians of different specialties, including cardiology, gastroenterology, traumatology, astromology, neurology, gynecology, urology, nephrology, and others.[77] Each doctor in the group has his or her own technician, receptionist, and nurses. The group was formed because a group of well-trained doctors wanted to work with each other. Dr. Compoy's credentials are an indication of the quality of doctors in this group. Dr. Compoy graduated from the National University of Buenos Aires in Argentina in 0971. His postgraduate degree is from the National Institute of Cardiology at Ignacio Chávez in Mexico City. He has three years of additional medical training at Mercy Hospital in San Diego, California, in the United States, has been a visiting doctor at Sharp Hospital in San Diego and Providence Memorial Hospital in El Paso, Texas, owns his own cardiology clinic, and is a staff member at Hospital San Javier where he is a member of the Scientific Committee. The doctors in his group have similar types of credentials.[78]

Dr. Ramírez works with a group of 30 multispecialty doctors such as ortho-pedic surgeons, internal medicine, dentists, gastroenterologists, plastic sur-geons, pediatricians, cardiologists, neurosurgeons, and others.[79] Dr. Ramírez's group of doctors has extensive postgraduate medical experience both in Mexico and abroad. Dr. Ramírez graduated from UNAM in Guadalajara in 1960 and did two years of postgraduate training in Phoenix and subspecialty training in gastroenterology at the University of Iowa. He has been the Chair of the Department of Gastroenterology, Chair of the UNAM School of Medi-cine, Associate Dean of the Medical School, and then Dean. Dr. Ramírez was the first member of the American Gastroenterological Association from Jalisco, is a member of numerous academic and medical associations, and has chaired many medical committees. Dr. Ramírez attends conferences in the United States at least twice a year and receives over 20 international medical journals a month. He is also the health advisor and the Director of Health Systems for IBM and the medical advisor to the American Consulate in Guadalajara.

This group of doctors decides together whether to admit any additional members. The two most important qualifications for joining the group, ac-cording to Dr. Ramírez, are having extensive advanced training in top train-ing hospitals in Mexico or abroad and having high ethical standards. The doctors jointly own a laboratory where most tests can be done. Some of the physicians in the group share medical equipment, materials, and sometimes office space and staff. An additional benefit to sharing materials is that they receive a 30 percent discount on medications and materials as a group.[80]

Dr. Sergio Zambrano Villa is an immunology and allergy specialist who works closely with two other immunologists.[81] This physician group is very specialized and has no formal relationships with other physicians. According to Dr. Zambrano, the Mexican economy and medical system do not allow the physicians to work together because there are a disproportionately large num-ber of doctors in Guadalajara and an irregular patient base. However, Dr. Zambrano has built a successful clinic largely due to his impressive credentials. He is a member of many international medical associations such as the Ameri-can Association of Immunology; American Academy of Allergy, Asthma, and Clinical Immunology; American In-Vitro Allergy and Immunology Society; and the Clinical Immunology Society. He continues to do research at the Uni-versity of Guadalajara in Jalisco, where he is a professor. He averages about four trips a year to the United States for conferences, additional training, and research. Each year, he attends workshops sponsored by the American Asso-ciation of Immunology and the Clinical Immunology Society.[82]

The average charges for basic services in Guadalajara and Chapala are relatively standard. A physician consultation averages N$150 to N$200, ac-cording to Dr. Carlos Torres and Herbert Rhoton, a retired American veteran who has been living in the Lake Chapala area near Guadalajara for over 30 years.[83] Some physicians throughout the Guadalajara and Lake Chapala region make house calls but charge the same office consultation fee.[84] Specialized services, however, have different price ranges. For example, Dr. Compoy, the American-trained cardiologist, charges US$60 for a complete heart examination and an EKG.[85] The examination includes a discussion of the patient's health status and a clinical examination where tests such as measuring blood pressure and heart rate and testing for arrhythmias and congenital heart defects are done. After the examination, the patient will either continue to have monthly check-ups with outpatient care if his/her condition is not critical, or, if the patient is critical, a cath lab (catheterization) and inpatient care will be recommended. Patients may be charged for additional services such as the cath lab, which costs N$2,500. According to Dr. Compoy, a similar procedure would cost around US$5,000 in the United States. Dr. Compoy sees most of his patients at Hospital San Javier, where he is a staff member and has access to all the high-technology medical equipment he needs, such as the cath lab. In addition, he feels that his patients have access to higher-quality equipment at Hospital San Javier, since equipment such as the cath lab is reviewed every six months and the engineers from the Japanese manufacturer service the equipment.[86] Dr. Parra estimates basic surgery for a peptic ulcer to cost about N$2,400 if he treats the patient at Hospital Del Carmen and N$1,600 if he performs the service at his office.[87]

Dr. Zambrano's costs also vary depending on the treatment required by the patient. For example, his asthma patients have to undergo four days of different studies and tests, such as antibody studies and X-rays, before he will prescribe any treatment. Treatment for two months, including medication, costs N$4,000 in Mexico while the cost could be as high as US$5,000 at Scripps Clinic in San Diego, California. Follow-up treatment can cost N$1,500 or more per year depending on patients' asthmatic condition.[88]

Most physicians see an average of 13 to 15 patients a day.[89] However, the number of American retirees that physicians treat depends on how directly connected a doctor is to the American Consulate and the American retirement communities. According to Dr. José González Alonso, he sees an average of about 12 to 15 new patients a month, in addition to his regular patients. Thirty-five to 45 percent of these are American retirees. The number often increases during the winter months because of the "snow birds" coming into Mexico.[90] (A "snow bird" is an international retiree who only lives in Mexico during the winter months, usually from November until March or April.) Most snow birds in the Guadalajara and Chapala areas are from either Canada or the United States.[91]

According to Dr. Compoy, he sees over 250 patients a month, of whom on average 25 percent are American patients from Guadalajara, Chapala, Puerto Vallarta, and Manzanillo. The Guadalajara and Lake Chapala American retirees are the majority of his American patients.[92] Dr. Zambrano sees one to two American retirees a week and about 20 Mexican Americans a month.[93] Dr. Ramírez averages about 60 patients a week, of whom two or three are Americans. Many of the American retirees learn about trusted Mexican physicians through word of mouth from friends or neighbors, the American Consulate, or American social groups, such as the American Society and the American Legion.[94] The Guadalajara office of the American Consulate has a list of physicians, surgeons, and dentists practicing in the greater Guadalajara area. According to the American Consulate, "this list has been prepared by the Consulate General for the convenience of United States citizens seeking assistance in obtaining medical services."[95]

Most patients pay in full for each physician visit or service received. According to Dr. Alonso, most of his patients pay in full using cash or a credit card. Some of his patients have a private insurance company that can be billed directly.[96] Payment plans or schedules do not really exist in Mexico. Capitation has been attempted with different informal groups but without success, according to Dr. Arturo Rodríguez-Toledo.[97]

Home Health Agencies

While home health care is a multibillion dollar industry in the United States, it is a unique concept being promoted by only a few fledgling operations in Mexico. Furthermore, while regulation and cost controls are being put into place in the United States, obtaining licensure to operate a home health agency is relatively easy in Mexico and regulations are minimal.[98]

There are several factors that may account for the lack of home health agencies in Mexico. First, there is a smaller presence of managed care organizations demanding lowest-cost services.[99] Second, there is a relatively greater supply of physicians in Mexico. This results in lower prices for home visits and other personalized care by doctors as opposed to nurses. Third, hospitals tend to keep patients longer in their facilities, resulting in less demand for short-term in-home support following hospitalization.[100] Fourth, it is possible to obtain live-in domestic workers who can perform household chores as well as nonspecialized medical assistance.[101]

There are two organizations providing home health services that operate in Guadalajara. The first provides temporary staffing services that include nursing. This organization provides mostly unskilled nursing care by home health aides (nurse aides called *quiradoras*) for extensive periods of time. This company generally charges 150-200 pesos per eight-hour shift, but prices can be as low as 80 pesos for eight hours.[102] The second organization, MediCasa, provides home health care services modeled after comprehensive services provided in the United States.[103]

MediCasa is a newly established home health care agency operated by

President Baxter Brown. MediCasa provides services throughout Guadalajara, Chapala, and Ajijic. Its main office is located in Guadalajara but it also has a new office in Ajijic. MediCasa continuously revises services offered based on the demand in the community. Although these services are subject to change, they are provided according to the model utilized in the United States. For example, patients are evaluated prior to beginning services to assure comprehensive and appropriate home-based care. Most care is provided by nurses who make visits lasting no more than 45 minutes, unless unskilled nursing services are requested. In addition, MediCasa is working with local hospitals to provide discharge planning services to assure continuity of care.[104]

MediCasa serves mainly Mexican nationals but also serves a significant number of American retirees. MediCasa serves between 38 and 70 patients at any one time and currently employs 130 full-time and part-time professionals who complete work equivalent to approximately 70 full-time positions. Like many U.S. home health companies, MediCasa relies primarily on part-time relief workers; the agency employs fewer than 30 regular full-time professionals.[105] MediCasa provides a wide variety of services, such as offering flu vaccinations in the winter and caring for elderly persons with respiratory ailments. In addition, the agency locates and leases medical equipment such as respirators and oxygen tanks, which are not readily available outside hospital and clinic settings. MediCasa is working to develop hospice services, discharge planning, and training of domestic workers to provide unskilled medical support services.[106]

Home health agencies compete against doctors' care, which costs approximately 150 pesos for an office visit and 70 pesos for a home visit. In contrast, MediCasa currently charges about 211 pesos for the first home health visit, where a physical assessment is performed, and follow-up visits cost 180 pesos for more than 45 minutes and 118 pesos for less than 45 minutes.[107] MediCasa has experience billing U.S. insurance companies for home care provided to retirees who have emergencies while vacationing in Mexico. However, there is concern that there needs to be compensation for the delays in payments that are common when dealing with U.S. insurance companies. The lack of economic stability, including high inflation rates, makes immediate payment more critical. Most businesses in Mexico, including health care, require payment at the time of service.[108]

Nursing

Nurses in Mexico provide care in hospitals, clinics, and in homes, the same settings as nurses in the United States. They provide care as employees of private physicians and as independent contractors. However, the level of training is not equivalent to the training provided to nurses in the United States. Nurses are often not considered "professionals" by either Americans or Mexicans living in the Guadalajara and Chapala region. Nurses, however, see themselves as professionals. They complete one, three, or five-year programs that can begin immediately after completion of junior high school.[109] (Currently, the trend is moving toward students completing high school before entering nursing programs.) Furthermore, nurses are working to distinguish themselves with specialties in much the same way that doctors and nurses do in the United States. For example, there is a great deal of prestige associated with being the director of nursing in an intensive care unit or specializing in surgical procedures.[110]

There is a wide range of salaries for nurses, depending primarily on the setting in which the care is provided and level of education the nurse has obtained. According to the director of nursing at Hospital Del Carmen, general nurses receive the equivalent of seven or eight dollars (about 60 pesos) per full-time day of work.[111] Nurses who are specialists are compensated about 70 pesos (about nine dollars) per day. Nurses LIC (licensed nurses with the equivalent of a Bachelor of Science four to five-year college degree) can make about 90 pesos (11 dollars) per day.[112] Such nurses are usually clinical directors of nursing.

In general, nurses are compensated least by clinics. They are paid better by private hospitals, and slightly more than hospitals when they provide home health care through MediCasa.[113] IMSS nurses are paid considerably more for their work in IMSS hospitals. This is especially true when their benefits packages are taken into account. Finally, specialized nurses such as operating room scrub nurses are very well compensated even in private hospitals.[114]

Nursing Homes

Nursing homes are a significant industry in the United States. In Mexico, however, most families care for their aging relatives in their own homes. As a result, there are not many facilities in Mexico that resemble the nursing homes in the United States. For persons who are not fortunate enough to have friends and family to care for them in their later years, there are homes for the aged. However, these homes are developed and maintained for the indigent and more closely resemble homeless shelters than U.S.-style nursing homes. Most people, including both Mexican nationals and U.S.-born residents, indicate that they would not consider placing a loved one in a facility such as this.

La Casa Nostra is a nursing facility in Chapala that more closely resembles a nursing facility in the United States. However, there are several features that make this facility and others like it different from nursing facilities in the United States. First, the Mexican facilities do not provide nursing care for their residents. The fees paid to the facility usually include only room and board.[115] Generally, these homes do not provide linens for the beds, towels, or standard medical equipment. In facilities such as these, the individual schedules his or her own nurses to come to deliver care in the facility.

Hospice

In the United States there are many nonprofit organizations that provide medical care and support for the dying. Some of these services are provided in private facilities (especially for individuals with AIDS) but most services are provided in personal homes. In Mexico, however, the hospice concept is considered new.[116] In the Chapala and Ajijic areas, where there are a large number of elderly persons, attempts are being made to initiate such services. In addition, there is at least one AIDS hospice in Guadalajara: Ser Humano is an eight-bed nonprofit hospice for persons with HIV. This residential facility is in need of many basic types of medical supplies and equipment. In addition, the prognosis is more serious for most AIDS patients in Mexico since only a very small percentage of patients can afford the recommended three-drug "cocktail" of medicines.

For those covered under IMSS, AIDS patients are segregated into a few hospitals, and one has been established for indigent AIDS patients. Care for persons who are HIV-infected is made more difficult due to community prejudice, the absence of medical coverage by private insurance companies, and laws prohibiting homosexuality.[117]

Pharmaceuticals

Pharmaceuticals in Mexico are reasonably priced and easily obtainable from local pharmacies. Pharmacists are licensed and individuals must receive training before they can buy and sell pharmaceuticals. However, regulations concerning pharmacy operations are not comparable to U.S. standards. For example, an individual with three days of government-sponsored training can buy and sell non-narcotic pharmaceuticals. A physician with three days' training can buy and sell narcotics. Pharmacists must obtain either a one, three, or five-year degree. Unlike in the United States, there are generally no hospital pharmacists or clinical pharmacists.[118] The maximum price for drugs is set by a national regulating board.[119] Pharmacies compete by offering discounts below this price ceiling, and many discount medical programs also offer discounts on pharmaceuticals. Many retirees take advantage of these savings. For sample pharmaceutical prices in the U.S. and Mexico, see Table 4.2 in Chapter 4.

Medical Equipment and Medical Supplies

Medical equipment costs are substantial in Mexico. Many people believe this is responsible for the quality-of-care problems in many hospitals and clinics. For example, medical equipment sold by Mexican companies, like oxygen concentrators (about $800 in the United States), generally cost about twice as much in Mexico.[120] In addition, many basic health care supplies can only be purchased in bulk, which many organizations do not have the capital to buy.[121]

Hospitals such as San Javier have indicated that in order to negotiate the most competitive prices from a wide array of competing medical equipment and supply companies, they have three or four employees whose full-time job is to negotiate and secure materials at the most favorable costs.[122] In other hospitals, equipment like endoscopes is often owned by physicians who lock them in personal lockers. They do not generally lend equipment, so that they can preserve their specialized-care market.[123] Local physicians indicate that medical equipment like endoscopes do not tend to lose value over time. Sometimes a physician can sell a piece of equipment after five years of use for as much as was originally paid for it. In Guadalajara, the "Baby Bird" (a children's ventilator) is being sold by physicians for two to three times as much as they purchased it for.[124]

Problems in obtaining modern, reasonably priced equipment and supplies would be minimized by the development of group purchasing agreements among Mexican health care providers. Frances Ortiz Schultschik has been working with health care professionals interested in developing group purchasing agreements. Although no formal agreements have been made yet, many professionals in the Guadalajara area have indicated an interest.

Sample Comments of Retirees Regarding the Mexican Health Care System

Retirees have a wide variety of incomes, education, interests, and health care needs, and likewise, they have widely differing opinions regarding how to meet their needs for quality health care services while they reside in Mexico. However, one sentiment expressed repeatedly by retirees was well-articulated in one respondent's survey: "[It] is a vast injustice not to receive Medicare when it is taken out of our checks. Service is much cheaper here than in the United States. [The U.S.] government should be happy about that!"[125]

Many retirees are very pleased with the quality of medical care in Mexico. They are particularly impressed by the amount of personal attention they receive from their physicians. Many retirees have been successful locating physicians who speak English and provide what they perceive to be good quality care at very reasonable prices. One gentleman told a story of needing a full EKG and stress test to check for a cardiac condition. The charge for the full service was only 170 pesos. What's more, because the necessary equipment was in Guadalajara, the doctor offered to drive the patient to and from the procedure for only 30 pesos more. One could not take a bus or a taxi for that small fare, and the doctor spent the time during the ride explaining to the patient more about the procedure.[126]

One woman tells the story of waking in the middle of the night in 1994 with what turned out to be a kidney infection. She paged her doctor at midnight and he returned her call within five minutes. Her doctor met her at the emergency room with an internist at Hospital Del Carmen. Since the doctor's office was only one block from the hospital, he visited her often. She told of how when she felt chilled the nurses gave her a blanket and then four nurses also bent over her in the bed to warm her. She indicated that the nurses were wonderful and that many employees in the hospital spoke English. She had a private junior suite with a private bath for US$69 per night, and when she returned home she received house calls from her doctor until she felt able to go out to his office.[127]

One woman stated that she had a tooth pulled out, a temporary bridge put in, and a bridge and partial denture put in, all for 980 pesos.[128] This dentist apparently has all the necessary equipment but maintains only an informal office in her basement. Apparently both the very wealthy and those on a budget appreciate the quality and cost-effectiveness of this particular dentist's services.

Other retirees are either wary of the quality of care in Mexico or are unable to pay even the relatively small charges to have procedures or checkups done in Mexico. Many of these retirees will wait to receive even minor care until they return to the United States once a year or so.[129] Some admitted that they had conditions that worsen considerably because they wait to seek treatment.[130] One gentleman was concerned that although he was supposed to get the battery checked on his pacemaker every three to four months, this would have to wait until he returned to the U.S. at the end of the year for his medical care.[131]

Many retirees were concerned about what they would do in the event that they or their loved one needed constant nursing care. A survey respondent commented, "[Medicare coverage] would be a help to have . . . if I needed specialized care, I would rather remain here."[132] They were concerned that if this happened under the current system, they would have to leave their homes in Mexico permanently. Most retirees expressed a great affection for their new homes and would not return to the United States if they felt that they could afford to stay and receive good health care in Mexico.

Notes

1. Interview by Lauren Lacefield Lewis with Norma Francis, Treasurer, The American Society, Guadalajara, Mexico, March 15, 1998.

2. Lake Chapala Society, *1998 Lake Chapala Society Membership Directory,* Chapala, Mexico, 1998, p. 3.

3. Interview by Olga Oralia Garcia and Monica Clear with Geraldine Cortez, Federal Benefits Director, American Consulate, Guadalajara, Mexico, November 6, 1997.

4. Ibid.

5. Interview by Lauren Lacefield Lewis with Shawn Godfrey, Editor, *Guadalajara Colony Reporter,* Guadalajara, Mexico, November 7, 1997.

6. Ibid.

7. Interview by Lauren Lacefield Lewis with Janet Levy, American retiree, Guadalajara, Mexico, March 17, 1998.

8. Interview by Lauren Lacefield Lewis with Shawn Godfrey, Editor, *Guadalajara Colony Reporter,* Guadalajara, Mexico, November 5, 1997.

9. Levy interview.

10. Fran Furton and Bonnie Pittman, "Retiring or Relocating in Guadalajara," Guadalajara, Mexico, November 1997, p. 1 (article in flier distributed to visitors in Guadalajara).

11. Ibid.

12. The American Society in Guadalajara, *Membership Directory 1997-1998,* Guadalajara, Mexico, 1997, pp. 30-31; interview by Lauren Lacefield Lewis with Norma Francis and Ann Smith, American retirees, Guadalajara, Mexico, March 17, 1998.

13. The Lake Chapala Society, "About the Lake Chapala Society," *1998 Lake Chapala Society Membership Directory,* Ajijic, Mexico, 1998, pp. 3-5.

14. From postings on the Community Events Bulletin Board at the Lake Chapala Society, Ajijic, Mexico, March 20, 1998.

15. Francis and Smith interview.

16. Service Directory for *El Ojo Del Lago,* vol. 14, no. 7, Ajijic, Mexico, March 1998 edition, p. 40.

17. Mexico Retirement and Travel Assistance, "MRTA Cost of Living Supplement, Spring 1997," *The MRTA Mexico Living and Travel Newsletter* (Spring 1997 edition), p. 23.

18. Francis and Smith interview.

19. Ibid.

20. Interviews by Lauren Lacefield Lewis and Olga Oralia Garcia with anonymous retirees, Guadalajara, Mexico, March 17, 1998.

21. Ibid.

22. Ibid.

23. Ibid.

24. Interview by Lauren Lacefield Lewis with Norma Francis, Treasurer, The American Society, Guadalajara, Mexico, March 17, 1998.

25. Ibid.

26. Anonymous Survey Respondent from Guadalajara, LBJ School Survey of U.S. Retirees in Mexico, March 15, 1998.

27. Anonymous Survey Respondent from Jocotepec, LBJ School Survey of U.S. Retirees in Mexico, March 18, 1998.

28. Anonymous Survey Respondent from Ajijic, LBJ School Survey of U.S. Retirees in Mexico, March 18, 1998.

29. R. Ham-Chande, "Aging: A New Dimension in Health in Mexico," *Salud Pública de México,* vol. 38, no. 6, (Nov.-Dec. 1996), p. 409; and S.A. Borges-Yanez, H. Gomez-Dantes, L. M. Gutierrez-Roledo, G. Fabián-San Miguel, R. Rodríguez, "Utilización de Servicios Hospitalarios por la Población Anciana de la Ciudad de México," *Salud Pública de México,* vol. 38, no. 6 (Nov.-Dec. 1996), p. 475.

30. Borges-Yanez et al., "Utilización de Servicios Hospitalarios por la Población Anciana de la Ciudad de México," p. 476.

31. Ibid., p. 481.

32. Ibid., p. 484.

33. Ibid.

34. Ham-Chande, "Aging: A New Dimension in Health in Mexico," p. 415.

35. G. Olaiz-Fernández, M. A. Lezana-Fernández, S.B. Fernández-Canton, R. Wong-Luna, and J. Sepúlveda-Amor, "Private Medicine in Mexico: The Results of the National Census of Private Hospital Units," *Salud Pública de México,* vol. 37, no. 1 (Jan.-Feb. 1995), p. 14.

36. Ibid., p. 16.

37. Ibid., p. 15.

38. Anonymous Survey Respondent from Guadalajara, LBJ School Survey of U.S. Retirees in Mexico, March 15, 1998.

39. Interview by Olga Oralia Garcia with Dr. Omar Aguilar, Director, Hospital Mexico-Americano, Guadalajara, Mexico, November 6, 1997.

40. Ibid.

41. Ibid.

42. Tricare Support Office, *Tricare Standard Handbook* (Aurora, Colo., September 1997), p. 156.

43. Ibid.

44. Ibid.

45. Ibid.

46. Ibid.

47. Ibid.

48. Interview by Olga Oralia Garcia with Martha Alcaráz Cruz, Director, Public Relations, Hospital Del Carmen, Guadalajara, Mexico, November 7, 1997.

49. Ibid.

50. Interview by Olga Oralia Garcia and Lauren Lacefield Lewis with Dr. Jaime Ramírez Parra, F.A.C.P., Guadalajara, Mexico, March 18, 1998.

51. Interview by Olga Oralia Garcia with Dr. Javier Michel Ochoa, Medical Director, Hospital Del Carmen, Guadalajara, Mexico, March 18, 1998.

52. Cruz interview.

53. Ibid.

54. Ibid.

55. Ibid.

56. Interview by Olga Oralia Garcia with Carlos Rodríguez Zárate, Administrative Director, Hospital San Javier, Guadalajara, Mexico, November 6, 1997.

57. Ibid.

58. Ibid.

59. Ibid.

60. Ibid.

61. Ibid.

62. Class presentation by Frances Ortiz Schultschik, Director, International Services, Methodist Healthcare System, at the Lyndon B. Johnson School of Public Affairs, Austin, Texas, February 17, 1998.

63. Ibid.

64. Interview by Monica Clear with Dr. Moisés Hernández Nuno, Hospital Administrator, Hospital Sharp Americas, Guadalajara, Mexico, November 7, 1997.

65. Ibid.

66. Olaiz-Fernández et al., "Private Medicine in Mexico," p. 17.

67. J. Frenk, L. Durán-Arenas, A. Vázquez-Segovia, C. García, D. Vázquez, "The Physicians of Mexico, 1970-1990," *Salud Pública de México,* vol. 37, no. 1 (Jan.-Feb. 1995), p. 22.

68. Ramírez interview.

69. Interview by Olga Oralia Garcia with Dr. José Gonzalez Alonso, Staff Physician, Hospital Mexico-Americano, Guadalajara, Mexico, November 7, 1997.

70. Cruz interview.

71. Ibid.

72. Ibid.

73. Aguilar interview.

74. Rodríguez interview.

75. Interview by Olga Oralia Garcia with Dr. Juan Carlos Órtíz, Physician, Guadalajara, Mexico, November 6, 1997.

76. Dr. Arturo Rodríguez-Toledo, "Informacíon Solicitada," Personal email to Olga Oralia Garcia, November 4, 1997.

77. Interview by Olga Oralia Garcia and Lauren Lacefield Lewis with Dr. Alfredo Compoy Diaz, Unidad de Cardiología, Cardiología Intervencionista, Guadalajara, Mexico, March 17, 1998.

78. Ibid.

79. Ramírez interview.

80. Ibid.

81. Interview by Olga Oralia Garcia with Dr. Sergio Zambrano Villa, Owner, Unidad de Inmunopatologia y Analisis Clinicos, Guadalajara, Mexico, March 17, 1998.

82. Ibid.

83. Interviews by Olga Oralia Garcia with Dr. Carlos Torres Lozano, Practicing Physician, Hospital Mexico-Americano, Guadalajara, Mexico, November 7, 1997, and Herbert Rhoten, American retiree, Chapala, Mexico, November 8, 1997.

84. Rhoton interview.

85. Compoy interview.

86. Ibid.

87. Ramírez interview.

88. Zambrano interview.

89. Torres interview.

90. González interview.

91. Ibid.

92. Compoy interview.

93. Zambrano interview.

94. Ramírez interview.

95. Cortez interview.

96. González interview.

97. Rodríguez-Toledo interview.

98. Interview by Lauren Lacefield Lewis with Baxter Brown, President, MediCasa, Guadalajara, Mexico, November 7, 1997.

99. Interview by Lauren Lacefield Lewis with Alejandro Siller, President, MediPlan, Guadalajara, Mexico, November 7, 1997.

100. Brown interview.

101. Interviews by Lauren Lacefield Lewis with anonymous retirees at the American Legion, Lake Chapala, Mexico, and the American Society, Guadalajara, Mexico, November 8, 1997.

102. Brown interview.

103. Ibid.

104. Ibid.

105. Ibid.

106. Ibid.

107. Ibid.

108. Ibid.

109. Interview by Lauren Lacefield Lewis with nurses and staff of MediCasa, Guadalajara, Mexico, November 6, 1997.

110. Ibid.

111. Interview by Olga Oralia Garcia with Marta Anilú Quijas Mata, Director of Nursing, Hospital Del Carmen, Guadalajara, Mexico, May 6, 1998.

112. Ibid.

113. Brown interview.

114. Ibid.

115. Ibid.

116. Ibid.

117. Ibid.

118. Ibid.

119. Interview by Lauren Lacefield Lewis and Olga Oralia Garcia with Emilio Zamudio, Director, Program Evaluation of Health Services in Jalisco, Guadalajara, Mexico, March 17, 1998.

120. Brown interview.

121. Ibid.

122. Interview by Lauren Lacefield Lewis and Olga Oralia Garcia with Carlos Rodríguez Zárate, Medical Co-Director, Hospital San Javier, Guadalajara, Mexico, March 16, 1998.

123. Brown interview.

124. Ibid.

125. Anonymous Survey Respondent from Ajijic, LBJ School Survey of U.S. Retirees in Mexico, March 18, 1998.

126. Interview by Lauren Lacefield Lewis with anonymous retiree, Ajijic, Mexico, November 8, 1997.

127. Interview by Lauren Lacefield Lewis with anonymous retiree, Guadalajara, Mexico, March 17, 1998.

128. Interview by Lauren Lacefield Lewis with anonymous retiree, Guadalajara, Mexico, March 17, 1998.

129. Interview by Lauren Lacefield Lewis with anonymous retiree, Ajijic, Mexico, March 17, 1998.

130. Interview by Lauren Lacefield Lewis with anonymous retiree, Ajijic, Mexico, March 17, 1998.

131. Interview by Lauren Lacefield Lewis with anonymous retiree, Guadalajara, Mexico, March 17, 1998.

132. Anonymous Survey Respondent from Guadalajara, LBJ School Survey of U.S. Retirees in Mexico, March 15, 1998.

Chapter 6
Tijuana, Rosarito, and Ensenada

by Marissa Quezada and Francie Kalunde Wambua

MEXICO IS AN IDEAL DESTINATION FOR MANY U.S. RETIREES. THE STATE OF Baja California, in particular, offers a peaceful way of life along the coast. Most important, the cost of living, including health care, is affordable for most retirees on a modest income. This chapter will describe the American retiree communities in Baja California, the health care system available to them, and the cost of health care.

Population

Rosarito is a small quiet beach town of about 23,000 inhabitants located approximately 30 kilometers south of the city of Tijuana.[1] It recently came into the limelight during the filming of the blockbuster movie *Titanic.* About 6,500 Americans live in this area. Many of the Americans in the Rosarito area live in trailer parks, such as Popotla. Others, the minority, live in affluent communities built especially for Americans such as Castillos Del Mar, Villas Del Mar, La Misión, and Rosarito Shores. Both those living in trailer parks as well as the affluent retirees must purchase propane and potable drinking water. Power outages are quite common, and only the affluent own backup generators to deal with them.

Ensenada is a city of about 300,000 inhabitants, located about an hour south of Rosarito on the toll highway. It is a coastal town with an economy based on tourism. A large number of Americans live in this area. One reason so many Americans move to Ensenada is to enjoy a higher standard of living than they were able to in the United States, since homes and utilities are cheaper in Ensenada. However, as in Rosarito, many city inhabitants must purchase water and gas from delivery services. Many residents from this area travel less often to the U.S. than Rosarito residents due to the time and money it takes to make the journey. They spend at least one and a half hours at the border and approximately $12 in toll payments for a round trip.

Accurately assessing the number of retired Americans living in Tijuana, Rosarito, and Ensenada proved to be difficult. Most retirees residing in Mexico receive their U.S. social security checks at U.S. addresses or have their checks directly deposited into U.S. bank accounts. Thus it is impossible to identify exactly how many Medicare-eligible recipients there are. One problem discovered when attempting to assess the number of retired Americans living in Baja California is that many U.S. retirees do not register or legally become permanent residents of Mexico. They are able to renew a tourist visa by returning to the border every six months. This skews the immigration numbers obtainable from the Mexican Office of Immigration. According to the November/December 1997 issue of the *Compañeros Gazette,* Mexican immigration officials recognize the difficulty in assessing and keeping track of the large numbers of Americans living in Mexico.[2] In response, they have begun checking various tourist camps to invite people to visit the immigration office.

There are various reasons these retirees do not register. According to the retirees interviewed at a Baja Camp Society meeting, attaining FM-2 (resident) or FM-3 (permanent resident) status is a costly and cumbersome process.[3] In order to attain an FM-2 visa an individual must pay 500 pesos per year for five years, after which one may apply for permanent resident status. Many of the retirees feel that 500 pesos per year is too great a strain on their fixed incomes. Moving from FM-2 status to FM-3 confers some extra benefits, but it is not required, as there is no limit on the number of FM-2 extensions that can be received. In the survey conducted by the LBJ School of Public Affairs in December 1997, 76.1 percent of the American retirees interviewed in Baja California said they are permanent residents of Mexico. In the same survey, the retirees were asked what type of visa they held. Of the 64 people that answered this question, about 8 percent said they held FM-2s while about 57 percent said they held FM-3 status (see Appendix C: Data by Question, Questions 22 and 23).

There are a variety of estimates of the U.S. population living in these areas of Baja California. Regarding Rosarito, one estimate shows 13,000 Americans and another estimates 15,000, many of whom live in Popotla, an impoverished area of the city.[4] Another estimate gives 6,500 Americans over age 50 in Rosarito and its associated colonias, including Popotla, Castillos Del Mar, Villas Del Mar, La Mission, and Rosarito Shores.[5] A senior staff member of the U.S. Consulate in Tijuana estimated Rosarito and Ensenada to have 50,000 retired Americans.[6] Another source estimates that there are 70,000 English-speaking people in Ensenada.[7] About 2,000 Americans live in La Joya Beach Camp south of Ensenada; most live in mobile homes without potable water or city gas lines.[8] An American retiree organization estimates that there are

100,000 Americans living from the Tijuana border to Punta Banda, 60 percent of whom are 45 years or older.[9] One source estimates that the *Baja Sun,* an English-language newspaper, has a circulation of 250,000 in Baja Norte and Sur (about 50,000 copies are printed each month, and it is estimated that each copy is read by about five people).[10] Though these estimates vary, one can see that there is a significant population of Americans in Baja California.

An additional difficulty was encountered when attempting to identify the number of Medicare-eligible Mexican nationals and Mexican Americans residing in Baja communities. This difficulty arises because these individuals usually do not live within the predominately American communities, and therefore are much harder to identify. In Baja in particular, many Mexicans have worked in the U.S. while they and their families lived in Tijuana. These Mexican nationals are eligible for Medicare without giving up their Mexican residence.

Average Income and Average Cost of Living

Many of the retirees living in Baja California have small, fixed incomes and live in trailer camps. More than half of the retirees surveyed in Guadalajara made less than US$25,000 a year (see Appendix C: Data by Question, Question 27).

According to the retirees interviewed, those on SSI receive US$485 a month. The average income is approximately US$1,000 per month for single people and US$1,700 for couples. The number one reason U.S. retirees said they moved to Mexico is because of the lower cost of living, allowing them to stretch their incomes further. A small one- to two-bedroom house in Ensenada costs about US$20,000 to $40,000.[11] A trailer park lot in the Punta Banda area of Ensenada costs about US$100 to $150 per month, while a trailer lot in the Estero Beach area of Ensenada averages about US$240 per month.[12] A trailer lot in a retiree community averages US$600 to $1200 per year, with water and trash pick up averaging US$30 per month and gas US$6 per month.[13]

Use of U.S. Health Care Services by Tijuana Population

In 1989-1990 the University of California-Mexico Consortium and the Population Council funded a study conducted by Sylvia Guendelman, D.S.W., and Monica Jasis, M.D., M.P.H.[14] The study attempted to measure the extent of Mexican residents' use of U.S. health services. A household survey of 2,954 persons was conducted in Tijuana, Mexico. Of the 2,954, a random stratified analytical sample of 660 people was used. This study examined the extent and volume of contact the Mexican residents have with health professionals according to sociodemographic characteristics, insurance coverage, payment methods, type of visits, and health care setting. The results of the study indicated that 2.5 percent of the Tijuana population have used health services in the United States. The largest proportion of those using U.S. services appeared to be older people, lawful permanent residents, and citizens of the United States who are living in Mexico.

Health Care System

Hospitals and Clinics

As is typical in many developing countries, there are many small three- to five-bed hospitals in Baja California. Before conducting field research in Mexico, the research team identified the major hospitals in Tijuana, Rosarito, and Ensenada that provide services to U.S. citizens and might be able to approach U.S. Medicare requirements. The following hospitals and clinics were investigated: Centro Médico Excel and Del Prado in Tijuana; Las Americas (which since closed) and Sanatorio Del Carmen in Ensenada; and the Red Cross Hospital, IMSS, ISSSTE, and Family Care Clinic in Rosarito. Three of these hospitals, as well as the Family Care Clinic, are privately owned. Sanatorio Del Carmen is owned by Catholic nuns, the Red Cross Hospital is a nonprofit, and IMSS and ISSSTE are part of the Mexican governmental health care system.

Centro Médico Excel

Centro Médico Excel in Tijuana has 30 beds, including three in the emergency room. Its average census is 30 patients per month. The daily room charge is about US$100, and Mexican insurance (Monterrey Aetna, Tepeyac, and Provincial) is accepted for payment, as well as some American insurance in emergency situations. The services offered include gynecology, pediatrics, ophthalmology, cardiovascular, general surgery, ultrasound, obstetrics, urology, emergency, pharmacy, laboratory, radiology, CT scans, and magnetic resonance imaging (MRIs). Handwritten charts are used for recordkeeping.[15]

Del Prado

Del Prado in Tijuana has 35 beds, including three for intensive care (ICU), two for cardiology ICU, three for surgery, and two in the emergency room. All rooms have a bathroom, closet, television, and telephone, and the hospital operates at peak occupancy. Room prices range from about US$135 to $150, and Mexican insurance and cash is accepted. Services include general and thoracic surgery, internal medicine, X-ray, 24-hour laboratory, pediatrics, gynecology, obstetrics, CT scans, cardiology, angioplasty, trauma, and ambulance service. Patient charts and handwritten notes are transferred to custom-made computer software for recordkeeping.[16]

Sanatorio Del Carmen

Sanatorio Del Carmen in Ensenada has 33 beds, including two ICU, two for operating, one for maternity, and one in the emergency room. The hospital averages 250 to 300 patients a month. Room prices range from US$175 to $350 per day, depending on whether the room has a private or shared bathroom. Cash, credit cards, and Mexican insurance (Provincial, Tepeyac, and Centro) is accepted. No American insurance is accepted for payment. Services offered include outpatient, maternity, emergency, X-ray, surgery, recovery, ICU, pharmacy, and laboratory (no specialty services are available). The recordkeeping system consists of patient records that are written and filed.[17]

Red Cross Hospital

The Red Cross Hospital in Rosarito has 28 beds, including five pediatric beds, two labor beds, one delivery bed, two incubators, one surgery bed, six emergency room beds, and one stabilization bed. The hospital serves about 2,110 people a month. Services offered include anesthesiology, dermatology, gynecology, surgery, and ambulance service. The recordkeeping system consists of patient records that are written and filed.[18]

IMSS and ISSSTE

The sentiment of U.S. retirees interviewed in the Baja California Norte area regarding IMSS and ISSSTE reflects a lack of trust in the system, doctors, and protocols. The U.S. retirees interviewed generally said they would not use these facilities. Retirees in Ensenada did express faith and confidence in the Mexican military hospital. The only problem regarding the use of this hospital is that retirees are required to pay for all services received up-front in cash. Most retirees are unable to do this given their limited incomes. The LBJ School survey results for retirees showed that no retirees in Tijuana, regardless of income, had purchased IMSS coverage (see Appendix D: Selected Data by Location, Tijuana).

Family Care Clinic

The Family Care Clinic is a U.S.-originated franchise located in Chihuahua, Toluca, Cancún, and Rosarito. The Rosarito Family Care Clinic opened in September 1997 and by mid-December 1997 had served 462 patients. According to Family Care staff, very few of the 462 patients served were Americans, even though the clinic has some English-speaking personnel. The clinic employees four doctors, three receptionists, three pharmacists, and three nurses. The clinic contains two regular exam rooms, an obstetrics/gynecology exam room, and an ENT (ear, nose, and throat) exam room. The clinic sees seven to eight patients per day and has a fixed fee schedule. Currently no forms of insurance are accepted, though the clinic has its own plans similar to basic managed care coverage, called the Health Administration Membership. To become a member, an individual may buy into one of three plans, which include free doctor visits, a 20 percent discount in the Family Care X-ray facility and laboratory, and a 10 percent discount in the pharmacy.[19]

The services offered by Family Care Clinic are pharmacy, X-ray, prenatal up to eight months, newborn services, geriatrics, free vaccines (provided by the government), and services for battered women (the clinic has an agreement with DIF, a charity organization supported by the Mexican president's wife, to provide free services to battered women). The clinic uses Mediplan software, created by the Latino Health Foundation in San Diego, for recordkeeping. The software is used for the fee schedule, coding, and to track patient care and bills.[20]

An additional service provided to Family Care Clinic enrollees is assistance in emergency and hospitalization cases. In such cases, Family Care sends its patients to two local hospitals in Rosarito: Louis Pasteur and Santa Lucía. Both hospitals reportedly have the ability to perform routine surgeries. Family Care staff described both hospitals as small, clean, good hospitals. Unfortunately, the retirees interviewed expressed no desire to receive services from either of these hospitals. In these cases, or more severe cases, Family Care transfers patients to Sharp in San Diego via the Red Cross ambulance service or aerostat helicopter. It is nine minutes to Sharp by helicopter.

Other Facilities

Additional hospitals identified in Tijuana but not investigated include Hospital de la Mujer y el Niño, Hospital Guadalajara, Hospital Notre Dame, and Unidad Quirúrgica de Urólogos Asociados. Hospital Notre Dame is the only one out of the four that is considered a "Centro Médico," with more than 50 beds. The remaining three are smaller clinics with fewer inpatient beds.[21]

Estimated Number of Americans Treated

The number of Americans treated by Mexican hospitals depends on the location of the hospital and the severity of the ailment. For instance, Centro Médico Excel and Del Prado, located in the Tijuana area, do not treat a significant number of Americans. This is because retirees in these areas can easily go to San Diego for health care services. The majority of the patients treated by Centro Médico Excel and Del Prado are Mexican citizens with private Mexican insurance.

Similarly, the affluent retired community living in Rosarito tends to travel to San Diego for health care services. There is no major hospital located in Rosarito aside from the Mexican Red Cross Hospital. A significant number of Americans are treated there, but approximately 15 percent of them are teenagers involved in accidents along area toll roads.[22] The American retirees who use the Red Cross Hospital come from the Popotla communities.

A larger number of socioeconomically diverse American retirees use the Mexican health care system in Ensenada as opposed to in Tijuana and Rosarito. This is because it is further and more costly to travel to the border to meet one's health care needs. Before the Las Americas hospital in Ensenada closed in June 1997, many retirees used its services. Ensenada retirees said that if they needed to go to the hospital on a nonemergency basis they would use local physicians who provide house calls or go to Del Carmen, but if they had to have a serious operation like cataract surgery they would go to the United States.

Retirees surveyed were also asked what they would do if they had to go to the hospital on an emergency basis. Those in Rosarito who opted to stay in Mexico said they would go to the Red Cross Hospital. Those in Ensenada who opted to stay in Mexico said they would use the General Hospital, Del Carmen, or the military hospital. The remaining retirees surveyed said they would go to the United States.[23] The hospitals most frequently used by those willing to go back to the United States (all located in California) are Kaiser Permanente (Chula Vista), Friendly Hills H.C.C. (Whittier), Sharp Hospital (Chula Vista), Mercy Hospital (San Diego), the VA Hospital (La Jolla), Scripps (La Jolla), and Balboa Naval Hospital (San Diego).[24]

Physician Network: Quintero Associates

Quintero Associates is an affiliation of 180 to 190 physicians. Currently, this affiliation is a network group, not yet solid in infrastructure. The associates have a joint venture with Medi-Plan Integral, a PPO in Tijuana.[25] Through the joint venture with Medi-Plan Integral, Quintero Associates intends to create an HMO, a first-class hospital in Tijuana with equipment such as a CAT Scan Doppler, and a medical center with doctors that practice nuclear medicine. The project is estimated to cost US$40 million in start-up costs. According to the director of Medi-Plan Integral, Dr. Piña García, Medilink, a company in partnership with Quintero Associates, will absorb the risk of U.S. liability and will offer a 20 percent reduction in Mexican medical rates.[26]

Regulatory Bodies and/or Agencies

The hospitals and clinics in Baja California are subject to regulation by the federal Secretaría de Salud. In general, legal issues in the Mexican medical community have increased. A system of government arbitration is used to decide the outcome for malpractice cases. Approximately 80 percent of these cases are decided in favor of the doctors. Most Mexican doctors do not carry malpractice insurance.[27]

Physician Qualifications

Physician qualifications vary with each of the hospitals and clinics. The minimum requirement is that they are Mexican board-certified while the maximum is that they are both Mexican and U.S. board-certified.

According to the administration at Centro Médico Excel, all four of their doctors are board-certified in the United Sates as well as by Mexican Consejo. Before doctors are hired they must be approved by Excel's internal credentialing committee and they periodically undergo standard peer review. The goal is to team U.S. doctors with Mexican doctors to provide the best service possible. Dr. Gloria Hernández, cardiovascular surgeon, is board-certified in the U.S., Canada, and Mexico. Dr. Hernández is a partial owner of Excel and sets a high standard for the doctors hired. In addition to employing high-quality doctors, Excel requires the nurses to receive continuing education and training at San Francisco State University. The goal of Centro Médico Excel is to have the same protocols as in the U.S. Dr. Hernández states that Excel is aiming for high quality control and that Americans have trained Excel personnel in proper equipment sterilization procedures.[28]

Credentialing at the former Las Americas hospital requires the doctors to undergo approved postgraduate training at a major national or foreign university as well as current council credential certification. Dr. Juan Velasco (a partial owner of Las Americas) is a member of the GMI physicians group in Ensenada, which contains 38 regular members and 10 "class A" members (similar to partners). In order to be a member of this physician group, the physician must be board-certified as well as meet current council credentialing certification. Del Carmen doctors and the Red Cross doctors are only required to be Mexican board-certified. All Del Prado's practicing doctors are required to be Mexican board-certified, and in addition, many of the physicians were trained and did their residencies in the U.S. Del Prado also makes a concerted effort to monitor the curriculum and ethics of their physicians.

The Family Care Clinic requires Mexican board certification as a family doctor. Doctors must then pass a separate exam given through the Family Care franchise. After passing the qualifying exam, and before the doctor is hired, the medical coordinator for the five facilities also checks the doctor's qualifications. Once a doctor is employed with Family Care he or she must participate in monthly continuing education classes. Doctors are responsible for staying updated on medical information by using SHARP conference tapes, literature, and other sources. In addition, the doctors attend 10 to 15 national meetings over a five-year period. The nurses at Family Care Clinic are trained in reputable universities and lab technicians hold a four-year degree in microbiology.

According to Dr. Sergio Quintero Ruiz, medical director at Medi-Plan Integral, Quintero Associates (Tijuana) plans to have a board that will verify credentials by mail. All doctors must be board-certified, and all specializations must be confirmed.

Pharmacies

Baja California Norte has many pharmacies. All the hospitals we visited had their own pharmacies within the facility. The prices of prescription drugs are generally similar at all Mexican pharmacies, since the government sets the maximum price allowed. See Table 4.2 in Chapter 4 for sample pricing of pharmaceuticals in the U.S. and Mexico.

Home Health Care and Nursing Homes

According to physicians, hospital administrators, and retirees interviewed, there are no official home health care agencies or nursing home facilities in Ensenada and Rosarito. There are also no listings for home health care facilities listed in the phone books for these areas. Home health care services are provided by independent doctors, but treatment is limited to house calls where basic health care services may be provided. Retirees may also obtain home health care services by hiring a nonskilled live-in assistant for approximately US$300 per month. Among the institutions interviewed, Family Care Clinic said they provide unofficial home health care services to patients on their plan at a 20 percent cost reduction.

In Tijuana, three so-called nursing home facilities were found. The Asilo de Ancianos María Rubio is a facility on the highway to Ensenada that charges N$800 monthly for *sala general* arrangements (large open rooms). No individual rooms are available. The second facility, Casa Hogar para Ancianos, also provides care in a *sala general* setting. The suggested donation for this charity is N$500 a month. The third nursing home is Residencial Bugambilias, which charges N$680 a month. These facilities all use open-area rooms and do not provide medical care, prescriptions, or essentials such as blankets or towels. Due to the lack of semiprivate or private facilities in Tijuana, the quality of nursing home care may be an issue for Americans used to a different standard of care.

Insurance

One of the prevailing problems encountered when serving Americans at hospitals such as Del Carmen is that many retirees seek services without having money or insurance. These retirees may have American insurance, or be Medicare-eligible, but these programs will not cover health care costs in Mexican facilities. The majority of U.S. retirees surveyed did not carry Mexican insurance coverage (see Appendix C: Data by Question, Question 11).

The medical facilities visited by our research group, with the exception of Family Care Clinic, accept Mexican insurance such as Monterrey Aetna, Tepeyac, Provincial, Centro, and others. The Mexican insurance covers all "standard procedures." International and American insurance is accepted in emergency situations only, and the treating facility must call and gain approval from the U.S. company prior to services being rendered. According to Dr. Velasco of Las Americas, "Many Mexican insurance companies offer a variety of plans that range from affordable to expensive. For example, plans offering no deductibles are very expensive, while a typical plan with a 20 percent deductible is priced within reason. In this case, a 20 percent deductible means the patient pays 20 percent of the total costs."[29] Dr. Velasco stated that he pays US$2,300 per year for health insurance for his entire family.

According to Del Carmen administrators, 25 percent of their clientele have insurance and the remaining 75 percent pay cash. According to Family Care Clinic staff, David Brown, the vice president of the American branch, is working on insurance being accepted at Mexican affiliates. The consensus among many health care professionals is that Mexican insurance is disorganized, bureaucratic, and maintains poor relations with the physicians. Many doctors spoken to expressed much interest in contracting with Medicare and providing services to Medicare recipients in accordance with Medicare guidelines.

Examination of Possible Cost Savings

Lower Cost of Medical Procedures

Following are some average costs of procedures received by Americans in Mexico. The costs listed include hospitalization as well as doctors' fees, and are in U.S. dollars.

- Doctor visit: $10-20

- EKG and consultation: $150-200

- X-rays: $200

- Complete physical exam: $350

- Appendectomy: $650

- Cesarean-section birth: $1200-1400

- Medically necessary facial reconstruction: $7,500

- Breast cancer treatment and prosthetics: $20,000

- Heart bypass: $40,000-80,000.[30]

Although the cost of medical care is lower in Mexico than in the U.S., it can still put a strain on a retiree's income. The majority of retirees interviewed (72.8 percent) said they pay cash for medical services received (see Appendix C: Data by Question, Question 3). In our survey, when 88 people in Rosarito and Ensenada were asked if they would use Medicare if its benefits were extended to them in Mexico, 71 percent answered yes (see Appendix C: Data by Question, Question 13).

Project Showing Cost Savings

While the research team was in Mexico, Dr. J. Marco Capucetti, one of the doctors interviewed, described a study he administered called the Calico Project.[31] In his report, Dr. Capucetti claims this project/case study is a good indicator of anticipated costs savings if Medicare eligibility is extended to U.S. retirees living in Mexico. The theory of the Calico Project was to prove to major third-party insurance companies that cost savings for medical management of U.S. citizens and non-U.S. citizens who qualify for U.S. benefits (such as workers' compensation) are possible through the utilization of Mexican health care providers, hospitals, and related services (laboratory, X-rays, nursing, etc.).

The five-year project was initiated in Ensenada, Mexico. Dr. Capucetti, the author of the study, and the Calico medical provider network (all Mexican physicians) began the management of workers' compensation cases through the California injured workers system and the State Compensation Insurance Fund. (The Calico Medical Network focused on primary medical surgical and hospitalization services, as well as contracted dental, chiropractic, and convalescent services for their U.S. patients.) Authorization for treating these injured workers was facilitated by the fact that Dr. Capucetti's prior working arrangement with the California system was as a licensed medical provider. Initially it was difficult to seek reimbursement from U.S. insurance companies for services rendered outside U.S. borders. But according to the report, the insurance companies assigned managers to each case, and once the assigned manager became aware of the author's credentials and license, authorization became easier to obtain. Once the apprehension about reimbursing for medical treatment in Mexico was overcome, the insurance company reported an average savings of 42 percent utilizing the Mexican network versus the cost of providing the same services in California over the same five-year period.

During this project, patients were asked if they were satisfied with the medical personnel, end result, quickness of procedures, rapidity of insurance reimbursement of medical services, and the hospitality of treating personnel. Patients were also asked if they would recommend or reuse these services. Overall, 80 to 90 percent of the patients were satisfied with the services received from the Mexican network. The Calico Report argues that the cost savings seen in this project would hold true in Medicare if coverage was extended to U.S. retirees in Mexico. The author estimates that the savings to the Medicare system would conservatively be between one to four million dollars per month.

Notes

1. Millicent Cox, *Demographic Atlas of San Diego/Tijuana* (San Diego: Padre Printers, 1995), p. 7.

2. Compañeros de Baja Norte, "Immigration Woes for Mexico," *Compañeros Gazette* (newsletter of the Compañeros de Baja Norte retiree organization), Ensenada, Mexico (November/December 1997), p. 1.

3. Interviews by Marissa Quezada and Francie Kalunda Wambua with retirees at the Baja Camp Society meeting, Ensenada, Mexico, December 14, 1997.

4. Telephone interview by Ann Williams with Michael Bircumshaw, Director, *Baja Sun,* Ensenada, Mexico, October 10, 1997; and interview by Francie Kalunda Wambua with Family Care Clinic staff, Rosarito, Mexico, December 15, 1997.

5. Interview by Marissa Quezada with Francisco Carrillo, Private Secretary to the Municipal President of Rosarito (Mayor Hugo Torres), Rosarito, Mexico, March 30, 1998.

6. Telephone interview by Susan Davenport with Juan de la Cruz, Senior Staff Member, U.S. Consulate, Tijuana, Mexico, October 15, 1997.

7. Telephone interview by Ann Williams with José Manuel Puig, Editor, *South of the Border,* Ensenada, Mexico, November 1, 1997.

8. Interview by Susan Davenport and Ann Williams with Nova Sampieri, Founder/ President, Punta Banda Scholarship Program, Inc., Punta Banda, Mexico, December 14, 1997.

9. Ibid.

10. Bircumshaw interview.

11. Ibid.

12. Sampieri interview.

13. Ibid.

14. Sylvia Guendelaman, D.S.W., and Monica Jasis, M.D., M.P.H., "Measuring Tijuana Residents' Choice of Mexican or U.S. Health Services," *Public Health Reports,* vol. 105, no. 5 (Sept.-Oct. 1990), p. 15.

15. Interview by Marissa Quezada with Gloria Hernández, Administrator, Centro Médico Excel, Tijuana, Mexico, December 13, 1997.

16. Interview by Francie Kalunda Wambua with Maria Luisa Reidel, Administrator, Hospital Del Prado, Tijuana, Mexico, December 5, 1997.

17. Interview by Ann Williams with Dr. Eloy Perez, Administrator, Hospital Del Carmen, Ensenada, Mexico, December 14, 1997.

18. Interview by Marissa Quezada with Dr. Francisco Chavez, Director, Red Cross Administration, Rosarito, Mexico, December 13, 1997.

19. Interview by Ann Williams with Dr. Abraham Bernstein K. Oidos, Owner, Family Care Clinic of Rosarito, Rosarito, Mexico, December 13, 1997.

20. Ibid.

21. Telephone interview by Susan Davenport with Pablo Schnieder, Consultant, Blue Cross/Blue Shield of Texas and Arizona, San Diego, California, April 5, 1998.

22. Elena Verduga, "1996 Statistics for Rosarito Clinic," *Cruz Roja Rosarito* (Mexican Red Cross newsletter) Rosarito, Mexico (November 1, 1997), p. 1.

23. LBJ School Survey of U.S. Retirees in Mexico, December 15, 1997.

24. Ibid.

25. According to Jim Austin (Owner of MediPlan), Safe Passage International Mexico, S.A. de C.V, owns the legal rights to the name "MediPlan," and Medi-Plan Integral is not to be mistaken with his MediPlan group, an international company based in Denver that has an HMO in Guadalajara and provides insurance. According to Jim Austin, there is also a PPO in Tijuana that calls itself Medi-Integral HMO, but this organization has no affiliation with Jim Austin's MediPlan HMO.

26. Schnieder interview. Pablo Schnieder stated that Medilink was no longer in partnership with Quintero Associates.

27. Interview by Francie Kalunda Wambua with Dr. Juan Velasco, former director, Las Americas Hospital, Ensenada, Mexico, December 15, 1997.

28. Hernández interview.

29. Velasco interview.

30. Interview by Francie Kalunda Wambua and Susan Davenport with Dr. J. Marco Capucetti, Medico Cirujano-Quiropráctico, Dr. John Zeffer, C.P., Prosethetist-Orthotist, and Dr. Juan Velasco, former director of Las Americas, Ensenada, Mexico, December 14, 1997; and interviews by Marissa Quezada and Ann Williams with Nova Sampieri and anonymous retirees in Punta Banda and Ensenada, Mexico, December 14, 1997.

31. The Calico Report (1993) reported on a five-year project. The study was authored by Dr. J. Marco Capucetti, a U.S. citizen who is a licensed physician in both the U.S. and Mexico and is qualified in industrial medicine (Q.M.E.). Dr. Capucetti currently practices in Ensenada, Mexico.

Chapter 7
Mexican-Origin Retirees in the United States and Mexico

by Olga Oralia Garcia

Tʜᴇ Mᴇxɪᴄᴀɴ Aᴍᴇʀɪᴄᴀɴ ᴇʟᴅᴇʀʟʏ ᴘᴏᴘᴜʟᴀᴛɪᴏɴ ɪɴ ᴛʜᴇ Uɴɪᴛᴇᴅ Sᴛᴀᴛᴇs ɪs growing steadily.[1] The number of Medicare and Social Security-entitled Mexican Americans and Mexicans with American residency is also growing rapidly (see sidebar for eligibility requirements). The utilization of Medicare benefits is not as widespread among those of Mexican origin.[2] This may increase the cost of caring for the old-age Mexican-origin population due to the lack of preventative health care. The factors influencing their underutilization may be related to language, cultural, or accessibility barriers. In addition to the high cost of high-quality health care, many Americans have not been able to keep up with the rising cost of living in the United States. An option for thousands of Americans has been to retire in certain regions of Mexico with a lower cost of living and greater access to personalized medical services. The Mexican American elderly population may start to examine this option for similar reasons.

Authors Kyriakos S. Markides and Sandra A. Block stated the following about the elderly Mexican American population:

> We are only now beginning to understand the special health and health care needs of the elderly Mexican Americans. Even though they constitute a small proportion of the Mexican American population, this proportion is rising rapidly. Better understanding of how health behaviors and related socioeconomic, cultural and genetic factors earlier in life influence health in the older years is much more needed, as are interventions aimed at improving the health of the Mexican American population in general.[3]

In spite of lower levels of health insurance and medical care utilization,

Mexican Americans have experienced decreases in mortality from both acute and chronic diseases.[4] The connection between low mortality and better health, however, is not clear.[5] The elderly Medicare-eligible population

---

Medicare Eligibility Requirements

- Generally, a person is eligible for Medicare if he/she or the spouse has worked in the United States for at least 10 years in Medicare-covered employment.

- The person applying for Medicare must be at least 65 years old and be a citizen or permanent resident.

- A person younger than 65 with a disability or with chronic kidney disease may also qualify for Medicare benefits.

A person can receive Part A at age 65 without having to pay a premium if any one of the following apply:

- Person currently receives retirement benefits from Social Security or the Railroad Retirement Board.

- Person is eligible for Social Security or Railroad Retirement Board benefits but has not yet filed for them.

- Person or spouse had Medicare-covered government employment.

A person can receive Part A when he/she is under age 65 without having to pay a premium if either of the following apply:

- Person has received Social Security or Railroad Retirement Board disability benefits for 24 months.

- Person is on kidney dialysis or has had a kidney transplant.

In order to receive Part B coverage, a monthly premium ($45.50 in 1999) can be deducted from a person's Social Security, Railroad Retirement, or Civil Service Retirement check.

Source: Health Care Financing Administration, "Who's Eligible for Medicare?", http://www.medicare.gov/whatis.html#Eligibility. Accessed: February 20, 1998.

Social Security Eligibility Requirements

• A person may receive Social Security benefits after he/she has worked in the United States for at least ten years or forty quarters. (Persons who turned 21 before 1950 may have had to work fewer quarters for eligibility.)

• The amount that a retired worker receives depends on the worker's earnings between the ages of 21 and 65.

• A person can also receive benefits if he/she is disabled before reaching the age of 65.

• A person can switch to retirement benefits on his/her own work record if these are higher than those received from a deceased spouse's record.

• The spouse of a covered worker is eligible for coverage at age 62.

If a person is currently receiving benefits and has children, additional requirements apply, such as:

• A child's benefits will stop a month before he/she reaches 18.

• A child can receive benefits until age 19 if he or she continues to be a full-time elementary or secondary school student.

• A child may continue to receive benefits after age 18 if he or she has a disability. The child may also qualify for SSI disability benefits.

Source: United States Social Security Administration, "Chapter 2: Becoming Insured," http://www.ssa.gov/OP_Home/handbook/handbook.02/ hbktoc02.htm. Accessed: February 20, 1998.

---

among Mexican Americans will surely grow rapidly, and development of cost-efficient and preferred retirement options for this population will become quite important.

Before reviewing the future of health care options for the Mexican-origin population currently living in the United States, some background information should be reviewed. Some of the items covered include the Mexican-origin population in the United States, barriers to health care services experienced by the Mexican-origin population in the United States, and the inclination to retire in Mexico. When looking at the tendency to retire in Mexico, emigration patterns and the current Mexican American population in Mexico are important factors.

Mexican-Origin Population in the United States

The Mexican American population will continue to increase at a faster rate than the United States population as a whole. The U.S. Census Bureau estimates that this population is growing at a rate five times faster than the national average.[6] Mexico was the country of birth for the largest group of naturalized citizens in 1994.[7] According to the Census Bureau's March 1997 Current Population Survey, 27.2 percent of all foreign-born residents are of Mexican origin.[8] A total of 7,017,000 foreign-born residents were of Mexican origin, of whom 1,044,000 are naturalized U.S. citizens and 5,973,000 are not.[9] Mexican immigrants constitute just over a third (37 percent) of the Mexican American population.[10]

Of the total foreign-born population from Mexico in 1994, 900,000 people were 45 to 64 years of age and 287,000 were 65 or over.[11] In 1990 the resident population of Mexican origin totaled 13,496,000, of whom 4,344,000 lived in the South and 7,824,000 lived in the West. This number included all native and foreign-born people identified as of Mexican origin.[12] Of the 31,195,000 U.S. residents who were aged 65 or older in 1990, 1,057,000 spoke Spanish or Spanish Creole and 62.3 percent of those spoke English "less than very well."[13] According to the 1990 Census, the foreign-born population in the United States from Mexico who are U.S. citizens with Social Security income numbered 165,789, and those with retirement income totaled 74,845. Of those who were not U.S. citizens, a total of 91,951 were receiving Social Security benefits and 42,524 had retirement income.[14] In 1993 the Hispanic elderly constituted 5 percent of the total 33.6 million Medicare beneficiaries.[15]

Barriers to Health Services for the Mexican-Origin Population in the United States

Some major factors that affect health care accessibility are differences in socioeconomic status, communication and language barriers, differences in eligibility for services, and differences in physical and financial access.[16] A national study in 1980 that looked at the needs of Hispanic elderly also outlined the specific needs for Mexican Americans in general and found that the discrepancy between use and need of health care is very high.[17] Cultural and socioeconomic barriers are some of the reasons that U.S. residents of Mexican origin who live along the border often use health care services in Mexico.[18]

Hispanic elders are more likely to express a need for health services but less likely to be aware of services available to them than their Anglo peers.[19] As one researcher has reported, "Even though the Mexican American population is still relatively young, it is growing rapidly but remains socio-economically disadvantaged relative to the general population."[20] In a study performed by the Mexican American Studies and Research Center at the University of Arizona, approximately 60 percent of the 489 Mexican Americans surveyed reported at least one health utilization barrier.[21] Of those encountering a barrier, almost 54 percent were actually prevented from obtaining health care for themselves.[22]

Access to health care is defined as having both health insurance coverage and a regular source of health care. Researcher Antonio Estrada has found that over one-third of those Mexican Americans with full access to health care encountered two or more utilization barriers. The main obstacles Mexican Americans faced were institutional barriers such as the cost of care, having to wait too long in the office or clinic, and delays in getting an appointment.[23] Cultural and language barriers have also prevented many Mexican-origin elderly from obtaining adequate health services. Even though attempts have been made to increase cultural awareness, diversity training, and other management methods so as to better understand how to serve minority elders, the underutilization of services among the elderly continues today.[24]

Cultural Barriers

The barriers to adequate health care for the Mexican American population have continued to exist despite advances in medical practices. Some attribute lack of health care to cultural barriers. For example, Dr. Max Offensburg of the East Los Angeles Doctor's Hospital, who practiced medicine for over 30 years in the Los Angeles area, believed that there is a "need for breaking away from the Mexican culture as far as health care goes. The Mexican people are not oriented toward health care. When they come to the doctor's office, they are *sick!*"[25] Dr. Offenburg's comments in 1973 touched on one of the basic problems of the Mexican origin population, a lack of early and preventive care. Therefore, rethinking the system of service delivery might help to meet the needs of a more diverse client population.[26] Some of the important factors dictating whether older Mexican Americans will use the services of physicians, including level of confidence, trust, and personal connection they have towards the individual physician, are affected by cultural factors.[27]

In order to better serve and to deliver high-quality health care to the growing Mexican-origin population, it is crucial to understand their health behaviors and practices.[28] Traditionally, Mexican families have taken the responsibility of caring for their own elderly family members. Mexican-origin elderly may have even more limited health care options than non-Hispanics if their children are less able to follow the Mexican tradition of caring for elderly parents, and if increasingly mobile families makes caring for the elderly more difficult.[29] "The plight of elders is becoming more serious as the extended family continues to break down under the inexorable pressure of internal and external migration, urbanization, and modernization."[30] "Adaptation to American cultural norms reduces the probability of Mexican children caring for their parents. As Mexican Americans assimilate into mainstream culture and adopt the lifestyle of middle-class Americans, these protective aspects of their traditional culture may be lost."[31] As the safety nets for the Mexican-origin elderly become weaker, their health care needs in the United States will become even greater.

Lack of Adequate Health Coverage and Affordability

The single most important barrier that continues to exist for the Mexican-origin population utilizing health services is affordability.[32] Besides being socioeconomically and educationally disadvantaged relative to the general American population, the Mexican-origin population also has a low rate of health insurance coverage. Approximately 32 percent of Hispanics of all ages had no health insurance of any kind in 1990, compared to 13 percent of non-Hispanic whites and 20 percent of blacks.[33] Even though an estimated 87 percent of the Mexican American elderly are covered by Medicare, this proportion is relatively low compared to the general elderly population.[34] Moreover, the lack of supplemental private health insurance and Congress' attempt to reduce Medicare spending will disproportionately affect Mexican Americans and other minority elderly groups.[35] Minority elderly such as Hispanics are at greater risk during retirement because of the lack of a secure supplemental income, such as a pension plan.[36] Moreover, it is estimated that 40 percent or more of the elderly poor do not take advantage of Supplemental Security Income (SSI) benefits for which they are eligible because of the social stigma associated with "welfare" benefits.[37]

Mexican-Origin American Population and Tendency to Retire in Mexico

Due to the growing Mexican-origin elderly population who are of limited means and are not receiving adequate health care, the likelihood of emigration to Mexico may increase and follow a similar pattern that American retirees have taken since the end of World War II. According to the Social Security Administration, the total number of Old Age, Survivors, and Disability

Insurance (OASDI) Current-Pay Benefits recipients in Mexico was 55,069 in December 1994. Of this number, 24,639 were retired workers, 1,773 were disabled workers, 11,078 were widows or widowers, 7,648 were wives and husbands of beneficiaries, and 9,931 were children.[38] These numbers are likely a significant underestimate. Payments to Mexico are subject to a 10 percent withholding tax, and an increasing number of retirees have their checks deposited directly to their accounts in U.S. banks.[39] In order to understand the likelihood of large numbers of Mexican Americans retiring in Mexico, emigration patterns of the Mexican-origin population, health care barriers, and other growing concerns must be considered. In addition, the growing American presence in Mexico may also attract a larger Mexican-origin retirement population south of the border.

Emigration Patterns

From 1980 to 1990, the amount of emigration to Mexico for the Mexican-born population was estimated to be 201,000. The number of yearly emigrants averaged 20,068.[40] Of all the foreign-born population, the total amount of emigration to their countries of origin was about 195,000 per year during 1980-1990.[41] In the "Work in the U.S./Retire in the Country of Origin" model, the probability of emigration at retirement depends on when the immigrants arrived in the United States. "The younger the age at immigration, the longer the pre-retirement time period over which non-pecuniary attachments to the United States would strengthen and country-of-origin attachments would weaken. Both factors would make emigration at retirement age increasingly less likely" for younger immigrants.[42] This model might hold true for Mexican immigrants. However, the U.S.-born Mexican American population might follow more of the trends of American emigration when it comes to retirement issues. Also, unlike most other immigrants, many Mexican immigrants stay in touch with their friends and relatives with trips back to their home towns and émigré groups formed in U.S. cities where they live.[43]

A Social Security report by Harriet Duleep suggested some conclusions regarding retirements benefits and emigration patterns:

- It is unlikely that immigrants entering the United States as young adults will work just long enough to be eligible for Social Security benefits and then emigrate.

- The longer immigrants reside in the United States, the less likely they are to emigrate.

- As the age of immigration to the United States increases, it is more likely immigrants will emigrate at retirement age.[44]

These theories are also supported by a General Accounting Office (GAO) study conducted in 1981 of 313 randomly selected beneficiaries living abroad. The GAO analysis showed that the average alien retired beneficiary abroad had worked the equivalent of 9.8 years of Social Security-covered employment compared to the average beneficiary in the United States, who worked the equivalent of 20.5 years.[45] In order to receive Social Security benefits, a person has to work in the United States a minimum of ten years, or 40 quarters, for those who turned 21 after 1950.[46] (See sidebars, pp. 106-107.) Note that it is possible to gain a year of eligibility for Social Security if one only works for a few months during the year in the U.S. The projections made by Social Security do not distinguish among emigrants who leave the United States upon becoming eligible for benefits and the native-born or other U.S. immigrants.[47]

Even though little work has been done on emigration, Duleep listed four factors she felt accounted for emigration when she assessed the role of emigration on Social Security's financial status. Of the current and future foreign-born populations, she felt these four factors accounted for the lower emigration rates:

1. People would be less likely to return home if the home country's economic, social, and/or political conditions were worse than the United States.

2. The lack of family and friends in the home country after such a long stay in the United States might hinder emigration.

3. Immigrants admitted as political refugees are less likely to emigrate for fear of political persecution.

4. "The lower the entry earnings of immigrant cohorts, the lower is the subsequent rate of emigration."[48]

The majority of the Mexican-origin population leave Mexico because of domestic and foreign (mainly U.S.) factors such as financial reasons and less for social and political reasons. Political persecution in Mexico is not as common as it is in some South and Central American countries.[49] Mexican immigrants have closer family and cultural ties to Mexico because of the relatively shorter time span in the United States, while each new generation born in the U.S. is likely to have fewer family ties to Mexico. The point Duleep made shows that earnings may influence those with moderate incomes to retire in Mexico because of the high cost of living in the United States. "A majority of the immigrants who emigrate do so within 5 years of U.S. residency, and about 80 percent or more emigrate within the first 10 years. Only 13 to 20 percent of the immigrants who emigrate appear to do so after 10 years."[50]

Duleep emphasized the need for further research in patterns of emigration in order to determine the ability to forecast Social Security's financial status.[51] An additional reason to increase research on the Mexican American population would be to make adequate projections for the utilization of Medicare.

Total American and Mexican American-Origin Population in Mexico

According to the 1991 Mexican census, Mexico had a total population of 81,249,645, of whom 9,276,433 were 50 years old or older.[52] Of the total Mexican census population, the Mexican state of Jalisco had 5,302,689 inhabitants, with 633,815 over the age of 50.[53] According to the 1990 Mexican census, a total of 340,824 of its population were born in another country, with 194,619 of these born in the United States.[54] Of the total number of foreign-born people in Mexico, 29,712 reside in the state of Jalisco and 23,718 of these were born in the United States.[55] Jalisco is one of the Mexican states with the largest number of American retirees.[56]

The Mexican American elderly population is more difficult to trace in Mexico because they blend in with the Mexican population. Although often United States citizens, they may have been born in Mexico. One way of determining the propensity of the Mexican American population to retire in Mexico is to refer to the number of people receiving Social Security benefits in Mexico and to evaluate the number of people remitting money to Mexico. The number of people remitting money to Mexico would point to the number of people who continue to have strong family bonds in Mexico. As Duleep points out, the lack of family and friends in the home country after such a long stay in the United States might hinder emigration.[57] A close connection with Mexican relatives through monetary support might increase emigration. In 1990 the total number of U.S. Social Security payments to retired and incapacitated workers and their spouses, children, widows, or widowers in Mexico was 59,528 with monthly payments of $18,305,000 ($219,660,000) yearly.[58] Even though it is not known how many of these beneficiaries were born in Mexico or are of Mexican origin, this "flow of money is an expression of the social process of migration between the two countries."[59] Even more, the amount of money coming into Mexico from the United States is a clear estimate of the number of people who continue to have close ties to Mexico, most of whom are probably of Mexican origin.

In 1990 a total of 1,903,000 Mexican-origin residents lived in the United States.[60] In 1989, 55 percent of temporary migrants and 43 percent of permanent migrants sent money to Mexico.[61] Some Mexican migrant workers are permanent residents or citizens of the United States with a close connection to Mexico. A survey conducted in 1988 and 1989 in three states in Mexico–Jalisco, Michoacán, and Zacatecas–consisting of 608 interviews by household with U.S.-resident children of Mexican parents indicated that 42 percent of migrants were remitting funds.[62] These three Mexican states also have some of the highest total distribution of remittance. In 1990 Michoacán received US$309 million, Jalisco received $240 million, and Zacatecas $104 million.[63] Some of the Mexican Americans from these states may be those that come back to retire in Mexico at least part-time.

The very low cost of living in the three states above is also a major factor when Mexican Americans choose to retire in Mexico. For example, Sarita is a 62-year-old Mexican American woman who has retired to Mexico with her 65-year-old husband who worked in the United States over 20 years. They live comfortably in a very small Mexican town, spending about 30 dollars a week. Becky is a 63-year-old Mexican American retiree who has lived in Mexico for over ten years with her husband, who is 71 years old. They retired in a medium-sized Mexican town after working in the United States for over 45 years. Some of their work in the United States was under the Bracero Program, an American program that contracted Mexican field workers during the crop seasons in the 1950s. José is a 65-year-old retiree in a larger Mexican town who retired in Mexico after working in the United States for over 25 years. He was anxious to return to Mexico to work his own land and to be close to his Mexican culture.[64]

In a medium-sized town of 8,000 to 9,000 thousand inhabitants in the state of Jalisco, an elderly couple can live comfortably on US$300 a month. In a small town of 2,000 inhabitants in Michoacán, the cost would be US$250 a month for similar arrangements, and in a larger city of 12,000 to 15,000 inhabitants in Zacatecas, US$350-400 a month.[65] Table 7.1 shows some average prices of various goods in three different-sized towns.

Rent is usually not part of Mexican-origin retirees' cost-of-living expenses because many own their own property, either inherited from Mexican relatives or paid for during their employment years while working in the United States.[66] For example, in the small town in Michoacán with an estimated population of 2,000 inhabitants, about 200 of the elderly population either receive Social Security and/or other pension income from the United States and own their own homes.

The Future of Health Care Options for the Mexican-Origin Population in the United States

According to a study performed by the Families USA Foundation, over 90 percent of U.S. residents who reported going to Mexico for health care were U.S. citizens or permanent U.S. residents. The vast majority of those who go to border towns in Mexico for health care would prefer to get their health care in the United States. However, the main reason for the utilization of the

Table 7.1
Costs of Goods in Different-Sized Towns in Three Mexican States
(in New Pesos)

Item	Small town in Michoacán (pop. 2,000)	Medium town in Jalisco (pop. 8,000-9,000)	Large town in Zacatecas (pop. 12,000-15,000)
Milk (per liter)	$5	$5	$5
Water (per gallon)	8	6	2
Bread (small loaf)	3	2	2
Beef (per kg)	35	36	35
Chicken (per kg)	40	20	20
Bananas (per kg)	4	3.50	3
Utilities:			
Gas (per tank)	100	89	100
Electricity (per month)	150	35	75
Soda	3	4	4
Haircut	25-30	15	20
Maid (per week)	250	100	150
Doctor consultation	70	50	50

Source: Telephone interviews by Olga Oralia Garcia with anonymous Mexican American retirees in Mexico, April 3, 1998.

Mexican health care system is the high cost of American health care.[67] In addition, many non-English-speaking Mexican Americans are becoming increasingly frustrated with receiving materials that are not in their native, primary language, materials that are not properly developed or easy to understand, and the lack of a sufficient number of bilingual medical assistants.[68] In response to the rising cost of health care in the United States, increasing numbers of American retirees living in Mexico have also chosen to seek medical services in Mexico.[69]

Many American retirees have pension plans, in addition to Social Security, that improve their standard of living in Mexico. As the number of Mexican-origin elderly increase and their pension plans improve in the United States, the tendency to retire in Mexico may also increase. The extremely low cost of living in some smaller Mexican towns and the lower cost of medical expenses as well as the opportunity to speak Spanish and live in the Mexican culture again might be the strongest factors contributing to the propensity of Mexican Americans to retire to Mexico. Many American retirees and Mexican Americans who previously lived in or near cities tend to retire in urban areas or very close to them. On the other hand, many Mexican American retirees who originated from very rural Mexican states, such as Michoacán, Jalisco, and Zacatecas, tend to retire to smaller pueblos. The different communities have something unique to offer to each group of retirees. The small pueblos tend to have a very tight-knit Mexican culture, where many of the elderly Mexican Americans feel more comfortable and secure due to the strong support system and the very low cost of living.[70] Given these factors, the tendency of Mexican Americans to retire in Mexico may increase as fast as the rate of Anglo retirees relocating to Mexico.

Notes

1. Frank D. Bean, Rodolfo O. De La Garza, Bryan R. Roberts, and Sidney Weintraub, eds., *At the Crossroads: Mexican Migration and U.S. Policy* (Lanham, Md.: Rowman & Littlefield Publishers, Inc., 1997), p. 137.

2. Ibid.

3. Kyriakos S. Markides and Sandra A. Black, "Aging and Health Behaviors in Mexican Americans," *Family and Community Health,* vol. 19, no. 2 (July 1996), pp. 11-18.

4. Jacqueline Angel, Ronald J. Angel, Judi L. McClellan, and Kyriakos Markides, "Nativity, Declining Health, and Preferences in Living Arrangements among Elderly Mexican Americans: Implications for Long-Term Care," *The Gerontologist,* vol. 36, no. 4 (August 1996), p. 466.

5. Markides and Black, "Aging and Health Behaviors in Mexican Americans," pp. 11-18.

6. Bean et al., *At the Crossroads,* p. 137.

7. Ibid., p. 133.

8. U.S. Census Bureau, *Country of Origin and Year of First Entry into the U.S. of the Foreign Born, by Citizenship Status: March 1997.* Online. Available: http://www.bls.census.gov/cps/pub/1997/for_born.htm. Accessed: February 22, 1998; and U.S. Census Bureau, *Economic Challenges Wane with Timing among the Nation's Foreign-Born Population.* Online. Available: http://www.census.gov/Press-Release/cb97-55.html. Accessed: February 22, 1998.

9. U.S. Census Bureau, *Country of Origin and Year of First Entry into the U.S. of the Foreign Born, by Citizenship Status: March 1997* (online).

10. Bean et al., *At the Crossroads,* pp. 117-118.

11. U.S. Census Bureau, *Country of Origin and Year of First Entry into the U.S. of the*

Foreign Born, by Citizenship Status: March 1997; and U.S. Census Bureau, "Introduction to the American Almanac 1996-1997," *The American Almanac 1996-1997* (Austin, Tex.: Hoover's Business Press, November 1996), p. 52.

12. U.S. Census Bureau, "Introduction to the American Almanac 1996-1997," p. 31.

13. Ibid., p. 53.

14. U.S. Department of Commerce, *1990 Census Population: The Foreign-Born Population in the United States* (Washington, D.C., July 1993), pp. 294-295.

15. Health Care Financing Administration (HCFA), *Profile of Medicare, 30th Anniversary* (Washington, D.C., 1996), p. 19.

16. Duran Bell, Patricia Kasschu, and Gail Zellman, *Delivering Services to Elderly Members of Minority Groups: A Critical Review of the Literature* (Santa Monica, Ca.: Rand, 1976), p. v; and Carmela G. Lacayo, *A National Study to Assess the Service Needs of the Hispanic Elderly: Final Report* (Los Angeles: Accurate Graphics, Inc., 1980), pp. 372-373.

17. Locayo, *A National Study to Assess the Service Needs of the Hispanic Elderly: Final Report,* pp. 391-392.

18. Families USA Foundation, "Going to Mexico: Priced Out of American Health Care" (Washington, D.C., November 1992), p. 3.

19. Lonnie C. Roy, Tracy L. Dietz, and Robert John, "Determining Patterns of Formal Service Use among Mexican American Elderly: Improving Empirical Techniques for Policy and Practice," *Journal of Gerontological Social Work,* vol. 26, nos. 3-4 (Nov.-Dec. 1996), p. 67.

20. Markides and Black, "Aging and Health Behaviors in Mexican Americans," pp. 11-18.

21. Antonio Estrada, *Beyond Access to Health Care: Institutional and Cultural Barriers Experienced by Mexican Americans in a Southwest Community,* Mexican American Studies and Research Center, report no. 25 (Tucson, Ariz.: University of Arizona, January 1996), pp. 2, 9.

22. Ibid., p. 9.

23. Ibid.

24. Roy et al., "Determining Patterns of Formal Service Use among Mexican American Elderly," p. 66.

25. Richard H. Davis, ed., *Health Services and the Mexican-American Elderly* (Los Angeles: Ethel Percy Andrus Gerontology Center, 1973), p. 14.

26. Bell et al., *Delivering Services to Elderly Members of Minority Groups: A Critical Review of the Literature,* p. v; and Lacayo, *A National Study to Assess the Service Needs of the Hispanic Elderly: Final Report,* p. 393.

27. Steven Lozano Applewhite, "Curanderismo: Demystifying the Health Beliefs and Practices of Elderly Mexican Americans," *Health and Social Work,* vol. 20, no. 4 (November 1995), pp. 247-253.

28. Ibid.

29. Angel et al., "Nativity, Declining Health, and Preferences in Living Arrangements among Elderly Mexican Americans: Implications for Long-Term Care," p. 466.

30. Scott Bass and Robert Morris, eds., *International Perspectives on State and Family Support for the Elderly* (New York: The Hawthorne Press, Inc., 1993), p. 10.

31. Angel et al., "Nativity, Declining Health, and Preferences in Living Arrangements among Elderly Mexican Americans: Implications for Long-Term Care," p. 466.

32. Ibid.

33. Ronald J. Angel and Jacqueline L. Angel, "The Extent of Private and Public Health Insurance Coverage among Adult Hispanics," *The Gerontologist,* vol. 36, no. 3 (June 1996), pp. 332-340.

34. Markides and Black, "Aging and Health Behaviors in Mexican Americans," pp. 11-18.

35. Ibid.

36. Angel and Angel, "The Extent of Private and Public Health Insurance Coverage among Adult Hispanics," pp. 332-340.

37. Ibid.

38. U.S. Social Security Administration, *Annual Statistical Supplement, 1995* (Washington, D.C.: U.S. Government Printing Office, 1995), Table 5.J11, n.p.

39. Interview by Olga Oralia Garcia with Herbert Rhoten, American retiree, Lake Chapala, Mexico, November 8, 1997.

40. U.S. Census Bureau Population Division, *Estimates of Emigration of the Foreign-Born Population: 1980-1990,* Technical Working Paper no. 9, by Ahmed Bashir and J. Gregory Robinson (Washington, D.C.: U.S. Census Bureau, December 1994), p. 12.

41. Ibid., p. 13.

42. Harriet Orcutt Duleep, *Social Security and the Emigration of Immigrants,* Program for Research on Immigration Policy, Urban Institute (Washington, D.C.: Urban Institute, May 1994), p. 16.

43. Telephone interview by Olga Oralia Garcia with anonymous Mexican American retiree in Mexico, April 3, 1998.

44. Duleep, "Social Security and the Emigration of Immigrants," p. 27.

45. Ibid., p. 28.

46. Ibid., pp. 14-15.

47. Ibid., p. 27.

48. U.S. Census Bureau Population Division, *Estimates of Emigration of the Foreign-Born Population,* pp. 9-10.

49. Frank D. Bean, Jurgen Schmandt, and Sidney Weintraub, *Mexican and Central American Population and U.S. Immigration Policy* (Austin, Tex.: The Center for Mexican-American Studies, 1989), pp. 21, 33.

50. Duleep, "Social Security and the Emigration of Immigrants," p. 21.

51. Ibid., p. 31.

52. Instituto Nacional del Estadistica, Geografia e Informatica, *Anuario Estadístico de los Estados Unidos Mexicanos, 1991* (Aguascalientes, Mexico: Impreso de Mexico, 1992), p. 230.

53. Ibid.

54. Instituto Nacional del Estadistica, Geografia e Informatica, *Estados Unidos Mexicanos Resumen General: Tabulados Complementarios Tomo I: XI Censo General de Población y Vivienda, 1990* (Aguascalientes, Mexico: Impreso de Mexico, 1993), p. 266.

55. Ibid., p. 268.

56. Interview by Olga Oralia Garcia with Geraldine Cortez, Federal Benefits Director, American Consulate, Guadalajara, Mexico, November 8, 1997.

57. U.S. Census Bureau Population Division, *Estimates of Emigration of the Foreign-Born Population,* pp. 9-10.

58. Fernando Lozano Ascencio, *Bringing It Back Home: Remittance to Mexico from Migrant Workers in the United States* (San Diego: Center for Mexican-American Studies, University of California, 1993), p. 60.

59. Ibid., pp. 59-60.

60. Ibid., p. 46.

61. Ibid., pp. 50, 54.

62. Ibid., p. 53.

63. Ibid., Figure 6.

64. Telephone interviews by Olga Oralia Garcia with anonymous Mexican American retirees in Mexico, April 3, 1998.

65. Ibid.

66. Ibid.

67. Families USA Foundation, "Going to Mexico: Priced Out of American Health Care," p. 6.

68. National Hispanic Council on Aging, "Latinos Encounter Many Problems with Managed Care," *Noticias of Hispanic Aging Issues,* vol. XIV, no. 3 (February 1998), p. 3.

69. David C. Warner and Kevin Reed, *Health Care across the Border: The Experience of U.S. Citizens in Mexico,* U.S.-Mexican Policy Studies Program, policy report no. 4 (Austin, Tex.: Lyndon B. Johnson School of Public Affairs, The University of Texas at Austin, 1993), p. 11.

70. Telephone interviews by Olga Oralia Garcia with anonymous Mexican American retirees, April 3, 1998.

Part 3
Extending Medicare to Mexico: Options

Chapter 8
Options for Medicare Coverage in Mexico

by Anjum Khurshid and David W. Lawrence

T HE FIRST STEP IN TESTING NEW ARRANGEMENTS UNDER MEDICARE OR MED-
icaid is to initiate the changes on a limited basis, which will permit
them to be evaluated and modified if needed before proceeding to
widespread implementation. The Health Care Financing Administration
(HCFA) permits Research and Demonstration projects under Section 1115 of
the Social Security Act. A formal research and demonstration (R&D) project
must be approved by HCFA. An R&D project is used to examine previously
unexplored options in Medicare or Medicaid. R&D projects can evaluate the
feasibility of new funding options, alternatives for provision of services, different strategies for overall policy examination, or other options. R&D projects
are powerful tools for HCFA to ascertain the effectiveness of various processes. When determining the outcome of R&D projects, one of the key factors is to evaluate whether expected results were achieved. Thus, R&D projects
must be designed in a manner that facilitates proper and useful evaluation.
The purpose for possible R&D projects proposed in this chapter and the next
is two-fold: first, the projects would examine the feasibility of providing health
care of reasonable quality to American citizens living in Mexico, and second,
they would increase HCFA's awareness of the growing needs of Americans
outside of the country.

As is demonstrated in the survey conducted by the LBJ School of Public
Affairs, people retire to Mexico for a variety of reasons, ranging from climate
to cost-of-living considerations. They do this despite the fact that they will be
sacrificing a fail-safe system of health care benefits. The purpose of this project
is not to determine if it is correct for them to expect to be treated like their
relatives who have chosen to remain in the United States; that determination
has already been made. The purpose of this project is to convince HCFA that
it is in the best interest of the retirees, HCFA's customers, that Medicare benefits be extended to Mexico.

The first step in evaluating the feasibility of extending benefits to Mexico is to determine that the need exists and that it will be cost-effective. In order to meet these requirements and demonstrate that this proposal is a valid policy initiative, an R&D project needs to be designed and implemented. Like the Medical Savings Account demonstration, this project must have clear goals and output measures that can be used to gauge the success of the project. Since the Mexican health network is different than the system in the United States, waivers will need to be requested to allow the flexibility necessary to make this demonstration possible. The R&D project regarding Medicare benefits for Americans retired in Mexico has many complexities and many uncertainties. But we have learned, through on-site research, that the communities of retirees living in cities such as San Miguel de Allende, San Luis Potosí, Guadalajara, the Lake Chapala area, and Ensenada have a definite need for improved medical coverage. Survey results indicate that American retirees in Mexico often live on incomes that range from US$7,000 to $35,000 annually. Thus, most of these people are not wealthy, and thus are very concerned with the cost of medical care. This demonstration will address their needs for Medicare coverage, and also examine whether they can receive reliable, reasonable medical care from competent health care professionals in Mexico and whether they should have to incur the necessary travel expense to return to the United States to use Medicare benefits.

The proposed research and demonstration projects are designed to provide necessary health care services and demonstrate appropriateness and cost-effectiveness. Both the beneficiaries and HCFA have to be satisfied in order for a demonstration to be successful. From the standpoint of the beneficiaries, any Medicare coverage would be preferable to none and would be appreciated. Traveling to the U.S. for routine medical expenses can be cost-prohibitive, and as a result, many retirees pay out of their own pocket for services in Mexico. A demonstration project offers options for Medicare that will provide an appropriate starting point. The options discussed include a full Medicare coverage study, a limited Part A and Part B study, a Part A study, a Part B study, an examination of Medical Savings Accounts, and implementation of Medicare Choice in Mexico. These options, however, are not mutually exclusive and are not the only feasible alternatives for demonstration projects.

Options

A variety of options for improving the situation should be explored. The complexity of the Medicare program and related factors, ranging from the populations to be served to the administration of the project, require exploration of several alternatives. All options are designed to demonstrate a possible cost savings when contrasted with similar services in the United States. The options are, therefore, designed to produce valuable data from which policy decisions can be made. Complete Medicare coverage implementation in Mexico as well as various combinations of sections of the program are all options. Some are clearly more comprehensive than others and some are more appropriate. These proposals cover some of the major options; however, we do not claim that these are the only options.

Complete Medicare

The provision of a complete package of Medicare services could be achieved in Mexico. This would be optimal for American retirees in Mexico, since it would make their health care coverage equal to that available to persons living in the United States. The major benefit in providing comprehensive coverage would be the increase in health care choices available to American retirees. Medicare, as it exists in the United States, could be made to fit and function effectively within the Mexican health care system. The combination of Medicare Part A and Part B would require a complex array of different types of health care providers. This would include generalist and specialist nurses and physicians, hospital care, trauma care, and home health care.

It would be necessary to contract with an entity to administer the program, to pay claims, and to provide oversight to ensure that necessary services are being provided with reasonable quality. This function could be achieved through a fiscal intermediary. If an entity external to HCFA were to provide this role, it would have to be familiar with HCFA's policies, the Mexican health care network, and procedures for third-party billing and data collection. HCFA has the means to track individual clients and their usage of Medicare services. The primary responsibilities of the entity providing administration would be customer service and ensuring that eligible persons are receiving the services required. Many hospitals in Mexico already provide billing services and enroll persons in their own health service programs. A more appropriate action would be to contract with insurance companies that are U.S.-Mexican joint ventures to serve as fiscal intermediaries. They are already familiar with both Medicare and with paying Mexican providers for services rendered.

Enrollment under this demonstration should be restricted to a small number of enrollees in order to permit effective evaluation of the program. By restricting enrollment to 1,000 eligible retirees from both Guadalajara/Chapala and San Miguel de Allende, a proper evaluation could be conducted. With 2,000 total enrollees, data collection would be more difficult, but the larger number would provide a greater number of observations and thus lead to more reliable results. The process of selection should be random and not based on a first-come/first-served basis. A random selection of enrollees based on the last digit of their Social Security numbers, such as using 2, 4, 7, and 0, would eliminate "competition" among eligible recipients. Once the pool of possible participants has been selected, a random process would determine which of those would be in the final 1,000 from each locale. And since in this case this is a completely add-on benefit and does not affect the beneficiaries' current Medicare coverage, it can be given to all selected persons and they can use it or not use it as they like.

Under this system, recipients would be able to travel between the United States and Mexico and use Medicare for health services in either country. A variation of this option would be to require beneficiaries to remain in Mexico for care, and not have transferable Medicare benefits. A "lock in" requirement, however, would likely detract many would-be recipients. Additionally, this would have a limiting effect on the Medicare program and would be inconsistent with HCFA Office of Research and Demonstration Theme Two goals of increased access to care and quality of care.

Limited Part A and Part B Study

A limited Part A and Part B study would entail full Part B coverage and Part A benefits in Mexico limited to emergency inpatient care only. Under this option, recipients are provided with greater opportunity to receive coverage than they would if they had to pay entirely out of their own pocket. This study would work in a manner similar to the full Medicare option. Differences would be present in the types of physicians that would have to be allowed as service providers. Since nonemergency inpatient hospitalization would not be covered by this option, certain specialists would not be regularly approved service providers. Trauma physicians, internal medicine physicians, cardiologists, radiologists, and other specialists who generally provide life-stabilizing treatment would be the approved service delivery personnel, along with requisite nursing and support staff. Part B services could be covered by a fee-for-service type of arrangement. Again, the administrative entity could be a qualified fiscal intermediary that had experience in Mexico.

Part A Only

A Medicare Part A study would provide options for recipients to receive inpatient hospital care. Since such a small number of survey respondents returned to the United States for either emergency care or surgical procedures, Part A coverage would have a positive impact on beneficiaries. Since inpatient hospitalization would likely be a less-frequently utilized option, limiting the program to 1,000 applicants in each area may not provide the necessary utilization data needed for a thorough evaluation of the program. This option would also be helpful in providing health coverage to tourists who are Medicare beneficiaries and obviating the need for special health insurance available to tourists traveling to Mexico. In this option, Medicare could agree to pay 20 or 25 percent of the cost for similar services in the U.S. and the beneficiary could pay for the rest out-of-pocket.

Part B Only

According to our survey results, over 75 percent of respondents indicated that they returned to the U.S. for diagnostic services, medical services, or routine services, all of which are covered by Medicare Part B (see Appendix C: Data by Question, Question 9). Again, due to the cost difference between Mexico and the United States, significant cost savings could be achieved in Part B. Both the federal government and the recipients could benefit, since health care is less expensive and travel costs would be reduced. Additionally, retirees in Mexico are often still paying Medicare Part B premiums. This option could operate in a manner similar to the other options that include Part B. Prospective enrollees could be randomly selected in order to minimize competition and bias, and claims and utilization review could be handled by HCFA or another entity. A wide and rather comprehensive array of services are covered under Part B, thus consumer choice would be increased.

The Medical Savings Account

The Medical Savings Account (as described in Chapter 2) would be an ideal option for recipients. Medical Savings Account (MSA) dollars are discretionary, as long as they are spent on qualified medical care. As of this writing, the Code of Federal Regulations had not been updated to reflect the law as prescribed by the Balanced Budget Act of 1997. Under a demonstration project, any Medicare enrollee participating in the MSA demonstration who was also retired in Mexico could use their MSA funds for any health care expense they chose. These patients would be able to display, in more immediate terms, how much less expensive the Mexican health care market is. They would be less likely to exhaust their savings account and more likely to build up a credit balance well above the deductible for the insurance policy while still paying for outpatient pharmaceuticals. The MSA demonstration could also be expanded with specific language to include other Americans living in Mexico. The evaluation of the MSA policy could also examine the effectiveness of the project with respect to persons in Mexico. This type of analysis would provide an immediate, side-by-side comparison of U.S. usage as opposed to Mexican usage.

Waiver Requirements

The Mexican health care system differs in many respects from the United States. Accreditation standards for doctors and hospitals are different, as is the culture in which medicine is practiced. One of the biggest indirect influences in American medicine is liability insurance for physicians and the threat of lawsuits for medical malpractice. This is not a real problem for physicians in Mexico, and most of them do not carry liability insurance at all. In the Mexican medical system, American standards will not be achieved overnight, or even in a considerable amount of time. Eventually, if HCFA is expected to approve Medicare for Americans in Mexico, adjustments will need to be made to make the Mexican system more compatible with the American system. But for the purposes of this demonstration, differences need to be settled by requesting waivers to implement the project. Waivers that deal with licensing standards should not be seen as lowering benchmarks, but rather accommodating a system that operates by a different standard and that has done so for many years.

The requirements of Medicare implementation that would need to be waived vary with the different options. However, some basic constraints would be applicable across all demonstration proposals. Essentially, these waivers would have to modify the demonstration to accept the Mexican health system as it is, and not insist on American standards as a requirement to receive American funds. The Mexican system would, however, have to demonstrate that although its standards are different than those in the United States, it is properly regulated by its own internal regulating agencies. These agencies would have to be considered legitimate entities and their policies would have to be accepted.

HCFA would have to allow many physicians with foreign training and certification to be qualified providers. Although some Mexican doctors have received training and certification in the United States, most have not. It would be costly and prohibitive to force American retirees to use only American-trained or certified physicians. Additionally, if requirements were built in that they must have American licenses, the numbers would be too small for an effective demonstration, and the real picture of Mexican quality of care would not be reflected. As the Mexican health care network system evolves, the internal certification and regulation of health care professionals will also evolve. Peer review organizations and similar groups could be given greater legitimacy. Such groups could also be provided with minimum standards of conduct by which physicians should be judged. Such entities would be ideal since it would allow HCFA to perform an administrative role, and not "micromanage" the program. A waiver granting Mexican physicians status as qualified providers would ensure greater options for retirees.

Hospitals would also need requirements waived, since many of them do not meet American building standards. A possible solution is not to demand changes in physical building infrastructure, like width of exit pathways, but rather ensure hygiene and cleanliness of the hospital environment, proper sterilization of surgical equipment and locations, and adequate emergency evacuation plans. Since licensing organizations like the Joint Commission on Accreditation of Healthcare Organizations do not exist in Mexico, such requirements for hospitals would have to be waived. The Code of Federal Regulations, in 42 CFR 482.41, explicitly states that a "hospital must be constructed, arranged, and maintained to ensure the safety of the patient."[1] Additionally, the CFR states that "The hospital must have written fire control plans that contain provisions for prompt reporting of fires; extinguishing fires; protection of patients, personnel and guests; evacuation; and cooperation with fire fighting authorities. The hospital must maintain written evidence of regular inspection and approval by state or local fire control agencies."[2] Such requirements would have to be amended for Mexican hospitals.

As mentioned in earlier chapters, home health is an area of service that is appreciably cheaper in Mexico when compared to the United States. However, because of cultural differences, the home health industry is not as developed in Mexico as it is in the U.S. In order to allow Medicare beneficiaries to take advantage of these lower costs, requirements for home health institutions would need to be relaxed. Home health aides in Mexico need to be allowed to perform home health functions without the levels of education and training found in the United States, and the functions that qualify as home health also would need to be adjusted. Many home health aides in Mexico do not perform the level of medical assistance common in the United States, but for the recipients, the services provided are just as necessary.

Aspects of Medicare policies that have been proposed to be waived would not undermine Medicare policy, nor would they undermine HCFA's authority. HCFA's Office of Research and Demonstrations (ORD) internal policies include requirements to provide improvements to health care financing and delivery and meeting the needs of vulnerable populations. A demonstration project examining Medicare benefits for Americans retired in Mexico is consistent with the ORD's mission.

Evaluation of Research and Demonstration Projects

Having outlined some options for conducting a research and demonstration project, the next logical step is to identify the means to evaluate its results. It will be necessary to have a research design that permits measuring the impact that this waiver has or is likely to have on the cost to the program, as well as changes in access, levels of satisfaction, and quality of care.

Research Design
For a research and demonstration project evaluating the feasibility of extend-

ing health coverage to Social Security beneficiaries in Mexico, several study designs are possible. Theoretically, there could be a pre-test/post-test research design, where the sample population is studied before the experiment to gather who they are, how they get their health care, how much they spend, and how often they return to the U.S. for getting health care (covered by Medicare); and then the same variables are measured after extending Medicare coverage to Mexico. From this comparison, we can arrive at the effects of this program on the use of health care facilities and also estimate its cost implications. This research design has some problems of internal validity, since the group selected for the experiment will be those who are willing to participate, leading to possible selection bias in the study. Such a design would also have to take into account that the attrition rate may be high since some of the participants might move back to the U.S. during the study period. Also, those who are very sick are less likely to stay in Mexico, and therefore the population of beneficiaries in Mexico may not include the sickest, highest-cost patients. It is also possible that the behavior of the participants may be altered temporarily to ensure success of the project, or their practices may be influenced by their being included in the study. This is known as the Hawthorne Effect, where the fact that people know that they are being studied affects the results of the study. There will be a question of external validity as well, i.e., would such a program show similar results if replicated in any other part of Mexico with a larger retiree population? On the other hand, simply providing this coverage to a population and documenting their medical care use, cost, and satisfaction can generate useful findings.

Another possibility is to have a control group and a treatment group. The control group will be a sample of the population that is not enrolled in the experiment and the treatment group will be another sample of the same population that agrees to be enrolled. Results from both the groups are compared to observe statistically significant differences in the two groups. The design works best if before the experiment the population is homogenous and the selection is largely random and unbiased. The beneficiaries may be picked randomly using data such as social security numbers or the first letter of their last names.

A third possibility is to use a case study methodology. The case study method is the method of choice wherein the phenomenon under study is not readily distinguishable from its context. It is also useful when the study cannot rely on a single data collection method because of a large number of variables. The U.S. General Accounting Office (GAO) has published a comprehensive methodological report entitled *Case Study Evaluations* that gives detailed operational advice for conducting evaluations of public programs.[3] The report emphasizes collecting evidence from multiple sources to enhance the validity of the case study. In this research and demonstration project, evidence about utilization and spending on health services may be collected from sources like interviews, direct observations, participant observations, and documents. A case study data file can then be created and results analyzed using various analysis techniques.

For any sort of evaluation, the instrument to be used will also be of significance. A survey of the sample using a questionnaire that inquires about health care expenditures and related details from beneficiaries might be the easiest, albeit not the most accurate, method to gather data. The Social Security Act allows HCFA to contract with certain public and private entities for the administration of the Medicare program. These entities are called "fiscal intermediaries" when they are covering Part A and "carriers" when they are dealing with Part B or Supplementary Hospital Insurance. If the program is administered through an intermediary, data on utilization and costs may be obtained through such an intermediary. A U.S. intermediary like Aetna Health Insurance that has experience working in a managed care environment as well as in the Mexican health system might be better equipped to generate such data. The advantage of having an intermediary is that it will be responsible for quality evaluation and payment for claims from the utilization in Mexico. The intermediaries would also be responsible for conducting medical review of claims to determine whether services were medically necessary and constituted an appropriate level of care. They would act as a deterrent to inflated claims or fraud. In any case, HCFA would be responsible for the evaluation or contracting for the evaluation with a third-party research group.

Indicators

The various indicators that can be used for the purpose of evaluation of the program include:

* quality of care,

* access,

* consumer satisfaction, and

* cost of health care.

Each of these will need to be defined and worked into the evaluation.

Quality Of Care

HCFA has two chief ways in which it measures quality of care for Medicare. The first is certification, where state or private accrediting bodies assess the quality of service. The second is monitoring through cooperation with providers. Some of the accreditation bodies include

- the Medicare Provider Certification Program (state agencies and private accrediting bodies assess whether fee-for-service institutional providers and individual practitioners meet the Medicare standards);

- the Clinical Laboratory Improvement Amendments (quality for all clinical laboratory testing is evaluated using these guidelines); and

- the HMO Medicare Contracting Program (assesses whether Health Maintenance Organizations meet Medicare quality standards).

The Health Care Quality Improvement Program (HCQIP) is the other way in which HCFA works with organizations like Medicare Peer Review Organizations (PROs) and End-Stage Renal Disease Network Organizations. These organizations work closely with providers to develop performance measures and improve information about Medicare beneficiaries' level of satisfaction. If a provider is certified by these organizations as following the Medicare standards set by HCFA, it is enough proof for HCFA that the provider can participate in the Medicare program. HCFA, in return, provides useful information to these organizations about Medicare health care utilization patterns and trends through the Medicare Quality of Care Surveillance System.[4]

The Medicare Provider Certification Program ensures that hospitals, ambulatory surgical centers, ESRD facilities, and home health agencies meet quality of care standards (also called "conditions of participation"). This certification process focuses both on the structural indicators and on beneficiary outcomes. The accrediting organizations include the Joint Commission on Accreditation of Healthcare Organizations, American Osteopathic Association, National Committee on Quality Assurance, Commission on Office Laboratory Accreditation, College of American Pathologists, American College of Surgeons, Commission on Accreditation of Rehabilitation Facilities, and the Community Health Accreditation Program, among others. The state survey agencies are usually the state health departments or state licensing authorities for health care facilities. These agencies conduct regular inspection of facilities to ensure that they comply with federal health and quality standards.[5]

The Peer Review Organizations (PROs), comprised of groups of physicians or physician associations, are paid by the federal government to monitor the care of Medicare patients in hospitals, ambulatory clinics, and HMOs. The PROs are contracted by HCFA, and hospitals and physicians are required to cooperate with PROs as a condition for participation in the Medicare program. Each state has only one PRO. The PROs follow the Health

Care Quality Improvement Program, which became effective in 1993, for Medicare quality assurance. According to HCFA, "HCQIP objectives are to: monitor and improve quality of and access to care; build a community of those committed to improving quality; communicate with beneficiaries and providers of care to promote informed health choices; protect beneficiaries from poor care; and create supporting infrastructure to make these achievements possible."[6]

The Mexican health structure does not have any of the above systems in place. Only through a gradual process of change and cooperation of the providers can these standards be introduced in Mexico. As mentioned above, HCFA has two main ways to measure quality: 1) certification, and 2) monitoring through PROs. Changes in the structure of health care delivery can be incorporated in the existing system in Mexico to ensure better service for the beneficiaries while at the same time protecting them from inferior quality health care. For the purposes of this project, quality checks would be made by the fiscal intermediary.

There are efforts to form hospital associations and professional associations in Mexico that could play the role of PROs or accrediting bodies for Medicare participation.[7] The peer review process is also being developed in Mexico, which could help work out the differences in standards between the U.S. and Mexico. Mexico has already established a national peer review board, which hears all legal cases of medical malpractice.[8] Regarding accreditation, the intermediary may get assistance from the various specialty boards in Mexico, as happens in the U.S. For general practitioners, a requirement of transcript verification and letters of reference from physicians involved in training the practitioner may be an efficient way of evaluating their credentials.

Access

Americans living in Mexico currently have the option to either use the Mexican health care system by paying out of their own pockets or to return to the U.S. to get Medicare benefits. Many Americans residing in Mexico rely on the Mexican system for their health care needs. A previous survey of retirees in Mexico showed that 43 percent of them come back to the U.S. for treatment each year, however.[9] The effect of extending Medicare coverage to retirees in Mexico may also be assessed on the basis of the ease of access to medical services. Greater access to health services may result in increased health spending by Medicare, but it may also achieve the desired outcome of better health for the beneficiaries.

Consumer Satisfaction

The purpose of the demonstration project is to look at the possibility of extending Medicare coverage to Social Security beneficiaries in Mexico, with the main object being providing better health care to American citizens through a system to which they have contributed for many years. It is therefore not unreasonable to evaluate the effort mainly on the beneficiaries' satisfaction. Of course, quality, liability, and other issues would also be taken into account. According to a survey, 94 percent of the American respondents living in Mexico indicated their willingness to seek medical services in Mexico if Medicare benefits were applicable there.[10] Medicare beneficiaries who live in Mexico seem to welcome the idea of Medicare covering some costs of health care in Mexico. It could bring a significant improvement in the quality of life of these American citizens who have worked to contribute to a system that was designed to help take care of them in old age.

Analyzing Cost in a Demonstration Project

One of the most important goals of a research and demonstration project for assessing the implications of providing health coverage to U.S. citizens living in Mexico is to show that it is cost-effective. In an era when the federal government is hard-pressed to cut down on expenditures on health care and to deliver more with less, cost savings is an effective way of getting recognition and acceptance for a new idea. Following is a discussion of some aspects of cost that might be incorporated into the evaluation.

Health Services

When measuring costs of providing health coverage to Americans living in Mexico, the first and most obvious criteria will be comparing the costs of the various services utilized: doctors' fees, hospital charges, procedural rates, and wages of paramedical professionals. The comparisons could be clearly made using the following criteria:

- fee for a visit to a general physician (primary care),

- fee for a visit to a specialist,

- charges for a one-day stay in a hospital,

- hourly rates for licensed nurses,

- rates for some common surgical procedures such as cholecystectomy, angioplasty, and cataract removal, and

- cost of common diagnostic procedures such as gastroscopy and bronchoscopy.

Assessing costs in the Mexican health system is not an easy task. Difficulties arise because of nonstandardization of services. Physicians usually have different sets of rates for different clients and are therefore hesitant to provide a rate list. This lack of standardization can make the assessment of actual costs of health services vary widely. It also leaves loopholes for fraud and abuse. The billing system of hospitals in Mexico also differs from that in the U.S. Hospitals may contract out any number of services and physicians can be owners of some of the diagnostic services used by the hospitals and bill accordingly. This raises issues about utilization of such services, appropriate comparable charges, and concerns about oversight.

Pharmaceuticals

Another important area where there is a marked difference in prices is medicines. Many people cross the border to get cheaper pharmaceutical products from Mexico, including many elderly.[11] Since Medicare does not cover outpatient pharmaceuticals, it is an important out-of-pocket cost for most elderly people. With the high prices of many medicines, paying for them becomes difficult for the poor and indigent elderly. If we know the average amount spent on pharmaceuticals by the elderly in the U.S. and compare this with what the same medicines cost in Mexico, we can evaluate the potential cost savings for the elderly who decide to live in Mexico. Reducing this expenditure by the elderly would not result in a cost-savings for Medicare directly, but it would prevent some people from becoming indigent and becoming dependent on the U.S. welfare system.

Cost of Living and Affordability

In 1992 nearly 80 percent of Medicare beneficiaries reported incomes less than $25,000 and 35 percent less than $10,000. One-third of the elderly relied on Social Security benefits as their major source of income.[12] It is thus relevant to examine the cost of living in Mexico as compared to the U.S. According to some sources, the costs of day-to-day expenses are 25 to 35 percent lower in Mexico than in the U.S.[13] Since health care expenditures are directly affected by standard of life, a higher living standard should result in better health status. Almost 62 percent of retired U.S. veterans surveyed in Guadalajara-Chapala described a lower cost of living as the primary reason for their residence in Mexico.[14] Don Merwin, co-author of *Choose Mexico,* a guide for retiring in Mexico, says that his book (published in 1994) claimed a retired couple could live comfortably on US$800 a month in Mexico. According to the author, the next edition will claim $600 a month will support the same lifestyle.[15] With a better standard of living, elderly persons will be able to afford more nutritious food and live in a better environment than they could afford in the U.S. Better climate is another factor that has favorable effects on the health of the elderly living in Mexico. Such a lifestyle in itself may reduce or prevent many health problems and bring a cost savings both to the individual retiree and the U.S. government.

Primary Care

Americans frequently travel from Mexico to get treatment that is covered by Medicare in the U.S.[16] Many of the conditions for which Americans come to the U.S. can be treated in Mexico easily and less expensively, and in many of these an early treatment in Mexico might mean saving the patient, and Medicare, costs for much more expensive treatment at a later stage. Social Security beneficiaries who cannot be reimbursed for their health care expenditures in Mexico may have a tendency to avoid health care spending until absolutely necessary. The managed care system widely in use in the U.S. is based in part on the principle of placing greater emphasis on preventive care to forestall diseases and resulting complications. Medicare coverage to these retirees may result in earlier diagnosis and treatment, thus preventing the higher expenditures that would be incurred at a more advanced stage of the disease if the treatment had been delayed until retirees returned to the U.S. for Medicare-covered services.

Increased Migration

Another dimension of this R&D project is to determine whether the number of Americans retiring to Mexico might increase if they could bring their Medicare coverage with them. First, we need to examine the main reasons Americans decide to retire to Mexico. We also need to discover the reasons that people do not move to Mexico who otherwise would. If noncoverage of health care by Medicare is a major reason why people decide not to retire in Mexico even if they wish to, then coverage will definitely increase the number of retirees to Mexico. As far as effects on costs, as increased numbers retire in Mexico they will take with them their contribution to the U.S. economy. Not only health care but other sectors might be affected by this trend. We need to take into account the fact that many people eligible for Medicare have reasons to visit doctors and/or hospitals regularly. If the amount it costs Medicare every year for certain elderly is reduced to one-third that amount because they can get cheaper care of the same kind in Mexico, then there is a definite cost-savings when people who are living in Mexico decide to remain in Mexico for treatment rather than return to the U.S. And, to the extent that they avoid becoming indigent, Medicaid can reflect substantial savings as well.

Administrative Costs

If Medicare was to cover the health care for Americans in Mexico, there are costs for supervision and administration that could offset much of the cost savings. Depending on the model selected for the demonstration, the cost of administration could vary considerably. A realistic cost-benefit analysis is possible by estimating these costs. One of the ways to assess costs is to find out how much Tricare Standard spends on administering its program in Mexico. The same process could be followed with several modifications to determine the approximate cost to administer this program. Tricare Standard deals with all the claims from abroad (including Mexico) through its intermediary, Wisconsin Physicians Service. There is a staff of only 30 people who handle all the claims sent directly to them by beneficiaries.[17] The administration of the program could be done through intermediaries in Mexico, which could entail a cost that is far less than administrative costs in the U.S. for a similar effort. Because enrollment would be concentrated in two or three cities for the demonstration, contracting with an intermediary with a Mexican base would make a lot of sense.

Practical Considerations for Evaluation

One of the most challenging tasks in evaluating a research and demonstration project is identifying measurable indicators to use for evaluation. A key question is how to first measure the utilization of services and health expenditures by Medicare beneficiaries in Mexico and then do the same for beneficiaries in the U.S. A problem arises because beneficiaries residing in Mexico will still be able to return to the U.S. to receive health services. For tracking utilization and spending in Mexico, a good way might be for the fiscal intermediary to gather this data. Such data is routinely kept by intermediaries in the U.S.; however, there might be some problems in gathering accurate information in Mexico due to differences in recordkeeping practices by hospitals and physicians. Most Mexican physicians' offices do not have computerized records, and most hospitals do not have cases organized according to DRGs (Diagnosis Related Groups), as is the practice in the U.S.

Interviews with people in the Research Data Assistance Center in Washington, D.C, reveal that it is possible for HCFA to track the medical expenditures of Medicare enrollees in the U.S. through a process of "cross-reference checking," at least for hospital utilization services. Each provider institution has an identification code; the first two digits of this code identify location, and Mexico is assigned "59." Also, each enrollee has an identifying number based on his/her social security number. If the social security number of a specific enrollee is provided to HCFA, they can use cross-reference checking to track the health spending and utilization by each individual.[18] With such data, the changing pattern of utilization and the cost of health services after extending Medicare to a specific population can be assessed accurately. Once the research and demonstration project is able to measure these changes, its results and conclusions will have a sound quantitative basis to evaluate the efficacy of this program.

Notes

1. Office of Federal Register, National Archives and Records Administration, Code of Federal Regulations, Title 42, Public Health, 42 CFR 482.41 (Washington, D.C.: Government Printing Office, 1991).

2. Ibid.

3. U.S. General Accounting Office, *Case Study Evaluations,* number PEMD-10.1.9 (Washington, D.C., 1990).

4. Health Care Financing Administration (HCFA), *Quality of Care Information,* http:// www.hcfa.gov/quality/qlty-1.htm. Accessed: March 7, 1998 (government information Web site).

5. Ibid.

6. HCFA, *Peer Review Organizations,* http://www.hcfa.gov/quality/qlty-5b.htm. Accessed: February 23, 1998 (government information Web site).

7. Class presentation by John Hilsabeck, Senior Vice President, Member Services, Association of Texas Hospitals and Health Care Organizations, at the Lyndon B. Johnson School of Public Affairs, Austin, Texas, February 24, 1998.

8. Class presentation by Frances Ortiz Schultschik, Methodist Hospital, San Antonio, at the Lyndon B. Johnson School of Public Affairs, Austin, Texas, February 17, 1998.

9. David C. Warner and Kevin Reed, *Health Care across the Border: The Experience of U.S. Citizens in Mexico,* U.S.-Mexican Policy Studies Program, policy report no. 4 (Austin, Tex.: Lyndon B. Johnson School of Public Affairs, The University of Texas at Austin, 1993), p. 33.

10. David C. Warner, *NAFTA and Trade in Medical Services between the U.S. and Mexico,* U.S.-Mexican Policy Studies Program, policy report no. 7 (Austin, Tex.: Lyndon B. Johnson School of Public Affairs, The University of Texas at Austin, 1997), p. 319.

11. Ibid., p. 24.

12. Margaret H. Davis and Sally T. Burner, "Three Decades of Medicare: What the Numbers Tell Us," *Health Affairs,* vol. 14, no. 4 (Winter 1995), p. 235.

13. International Global Report, "Many Seek American Dream Outside America," *Christian Science Monitor* (March 19, 1997), p. 9.

14. Warner and Reed, *Health Care across the Border: The Experience of U.S. Citizens in Mexico,* p. 223.

15. International Global Report, "Many Seek American Dream Outside America," p. 9.

16. Warner, *NAFTA and Trade in Medical Services between the U.S. and Mexico,* p. 319.

17. Telephone interview by Amy Sprague with unidentified claims processor, Wisconsin Physicians Service, Madison, Wisconsin, March 23, 1998.

18. Telephone interview by Anjum Khurshid with Wei Chung Yang, Research Data Assistance Center, Washington, D.C., April 2, 1998.

Chapter 9
Extending Medicare to Northern Baja California

by Susan Davenport and Ann Williams

A S EVIDENCED BY THE NORTHERN BAJA CALIFORNIA CASE STUDY IN CHAP-
ter 6, a significant number of Medicare recipients and Medicare-eli
gible persons reside in the Northern Baja California area. Extending
Medicare benefits to this area would prove advantageous to both recipients
and to the Health Care Financing Administration (HCFA). With the advent
of Medicare Choices and Medical Savings Accounts in the Balanced Budget
Act of 1997, the stage is set for beneficiaries to choose the health coverage
that best suits their needs and for providers to develop more innovative Medicare plans. The goal of this chapter is to examine alternative methods for
making Medicare portable to Northern Baja California and to present strategies for developing Medicare risk HMOs to serve residents of Northern Baja.
By outlining both developmental and structural issues, we hope to generate
dialogue and action among companies or organizations positioned to launch
Medicare coverage in Northern Baja California.

Existing Plans and Providers

Medicare Health Maintenance Organizations
in San Diego and Imperial Counties
According to a HCFA informational pamphlet, nine HMOs had contracts
with Medicare in San Diego and Imperial counties in May 1997. Many of the
plans provide additional benefits at no charge, such as annual physicals, prescription drugs, dental care, hearing aids, and eyeglasses. Most of the plans
have "lock-in" provisions that do not allow recipients to seek services outside
the plan except in cases of emergency. In a section dedicated to explaining
the characteristics of HMOs, the pamphlet explicitly advises recipients who
travel frequently to consider choosing a fee-for-service plan over an HMO.[1]

A similar HCFA booklet for Medicare recipients explains in detail the differences between fee-for-service and managed care plans. Under the fee-for-service system, Medicare recipients choose any licensed physician or provider. Medicare pays the provider a fee each time a service is used. The Medicare recipient is responsible for deductibles and coinsurance of 20 percent. Medicare recipients can avoid out-of-pocket costs by purchasing Medigap insurance, which covers some of the payment gaps in Medicare fee-for-service coverage.[2]

Requirements to enroll in a Medicare HMO include current enrollment and continued payment of monthly premiums for Part B, neither current medical determination of end-stage renal disease or elected hospice care, and residence within the area in which the plan has a Medicare contract to provide services.[3]

HCFA advises recipients to consider the differences between risk plans and cost plans. Most importantly, risk plans require recipients to receive all covered care through the plan or plan referrals. Recipients receiving care outside the plan must pay the entire bill out-of-pocket. Enrollees who are *temporarily* away from the plan's service area may often access emergency services for a small copayment. Risk HMOs sometimes offer a "point-of-service" (POS) option that allows enrollees to receive service outside the plan but requires them to pay at least 20 percent of the charges.[4]

Cost plans do not have "lock-in" requirements. Recipients may choose to seek medical care from the HMO's network of health care providers or from outside the plan. In this case, beneficiaries pay coinsurance and deductibles in a fee-for-service arrangement with Medicare. In *Medicare Managed Care,* HCFA advises recipients who travel frequently to consider a cost plan for coverage.[5]

As indicated in Table 9.1, Medicare HMOs in San Diego and Imperial counties offer emergency service worldwide. This is an additional benefit for those enrolled in HMOs. Normally, Medicare does not pay for health care obtained outside the United States and its territories, except under the specific circumstances described in Chapter 2. Table 9.1 shows the Medicare HMOs offered in San Diego and Imperial counties and outlines some of their features.

Hospitals and Provider Networks in Northern Baja California

Northern Baja California, which is considered as extending from Tijuana in the north to Punta Banda in the south for our purposes, has several physician networks and a fair number of hospitals and clinics. As mentioned previously, many small clinics and hospitals with ten or fewer beds exist in this area. The major hospitals and physician networks studied are described in detail in Chapter 6.

Table 9.1
Medicare HMOs in San Diego and Imperial Counties

Plan	Monthly Premium (1998)	Emergency Worldwide Coverage	Point Of Service (POS) Option	Prescription Drug Benefit
Traditional Medicare	Part B: $43.80	not covered	not applicable	not covered
Blue Cross Senior Secure (Blue Cross of California)	Part B: $43.80	$20; waived if admitted	$25 physician office visit to select physicians (up to 3 visits per year)	N/A
Senior Plan (California Care)	Part B: $43.80	N/A	N/A	included
Health Care for Seniors (Cigna)	Part B: $43.80	$25; waived if admitted	N/A	included
Senior Plan (FHP)	Part B: $43.80	$25; waived if admitted	N/A	included
Senior Value (Foundation Health)	Part B: $43.80	$35; waived if admitted	N/A	included
Seniority Plus (Health Net)	Part B: $43.80	$20; waived if admitted	N/A	included
Senior Advantage (Kaiser)	Part B: $43.80	no charge	N/A	included
Senior Horizons (Pacificare)	Part B: $43.80	$20; waived if admitted	N/A	included
Senior Care (Prudential)	Part B: $43.80	$35; waived if admitted	N/A	included

Source: Health Care Financing Administration, *Health Maintenance Organization (HMO) 1997 Benefits Comparison–Southern California* (Washington, D.C., May 1997), n.p.

Selected Cross-Border Collaborations

The San Diego-Tijuana border area has a history of cross-border collaborations in health care. Agribusiness companies have used the Mexican health care system for many years to provide medical plans to workers living in the United States and Mexico.

The Western Growers Association has offered health care plans in Mexico to workers for over 15 years. During the last eight years, it has operated its own Preferred Provider Organization (PPO) in Mexico. By making it significantly less expensive for employees to seek health care in Mexico, the association encourages use of the Mexican PPO and saves money on the overall plan. While employees seeking care in the United States pay a deductible and coinsurance of 20 percent, those visiting doctors or hospitals in Mexico pay only US$2.50 per visit. Of the 70,000 workers covered in 1995, 80 percent were United States residents and 20 percent were workers' dependents residing in Mexico. About 10,000, or 14 percent, of the total enrollees received their medical services in Mexico.

In 1987, Frontera Health Services, a Portland-based insurance company, and three Mexican physicians entered into a partnership to provide self-insured health care programs to U.S. companies employing Mexican residents or whose employees have dependents living in Mexico. Frontera negotiated contracts with eight hospitals and 125 doctors in Tijuana and Mexicali who agreed to a fixed fee-for-service arrangement with discounts based on increased patient flow. Since that time, Frontera has begun to offer fully insured programs. In 1995 the company had contracts with physicians, hospitals, clinics, and pharmacies in Tijuana, Mexicali, and San Luis Río Colorado.[6]

Most recently, Aetna/U.S. Healthcare has partnered with Seguros Monterrey Aetna and Meximed to market HMO coverage in California that provides benefits in Mexico. Aetna sells plans in the United States for coverage with a Seguros Monterrey PPO in Tijuana. This coverage is sold to employer groups, not individuals, and usually includes employees' dependents living in Mexico. Meximed handles the administration of the plan. The network is licensed in Mexico and licensed in the U.S. through an informational filing with the California Department of Corporations. The PPO network in Tijuana has 16 primary care physicians, 45 specialists, and four hospitals: Unidad Quirúrgica Plaza, Hospital de la Mujer, Hospital Guadalajara, and Hospital Notre Dame.[7]

Options for Medicare Coverage in Northern Baja California

Risk HMO

Probably the most attractive option for providing coverage to Medicare recipients residing in Northern Baja would be the development of choices between separate HMO networks for Medicare beneficiaries administered by a San Diego risk HMO. The HMO networks would cover all Medicare services (Parts A and B) and could offer a Preferred Provider Organization (PPO) or HMO option in San Diego and Imperial counties in addition to coverage in Mexico. To provide appropriate competition and to avoid "creaming," it would probably be best to offer choices of at least two HMOs with some oversight or separation of marketing and quality assessment. This type of risk HMO model with capitation has the following advantages:

- The provider infrastructure in Northern Baja California could easily support managed care networks for Medicare beneficiaries.

- Risk HMOs provide more services. As noted in the previous section, many HMOs offer full Part A and B coverage as well as prescription benefits and preventive care on a routine basis.

- The risk HMO allows for more administrative flexibility. HCFA would reimburse a U.S. administrator with one monthly payment as opposed to sending numerous payments each month to providers in the traditional fee-for-service model.

- An HMO administered by an experienced San Diego risk HMO would no doubt pay providers on time. Physicians and hospitals in the Baja area complain about slow reimbursement from insurance companies–some hospitals now refuse to accept Mexican health insurance for this reason.

Fee-for-Service

As another alternative for providing Medicare coverage to Baja California residents, extending fee-for-service coverage to the area would be relatively simple. The system would function exactly as it does in the United States, with the extension of provider coverage through Northern Baja California instead of stopping at the U.S. border. HCFA would select and designate certain Mexican physicians and hospitals as official providers and pay them an agreed-upon fee each time they served a Medicare recipient. The Medicare recipient would be responsible for deductibles and coinsurance of 20 percent and could purchase Medigap insurance to cover some out-of-pocket costs.

The major advantages of this model include coverage for the Medicare-eligible population in Northern Baja California and significant savings for HCFA. Due to the proximity of San Diego to the northern Baja area, most Medicare recipients currently avoid high out-of-pocket costs by visiting San Diego for more expensive, Medicare-covered services. By setting fees in Northern Baja based on Mexico's lower health care costs and allowing Northern Baja residents to visit Mexican providers, HCFA could realize substantial savings.

Preferred Provider Organization (PPO) in San Diego or Imperial Counties

As mentioned above, the California HMO administering the Northern Baja

HMO network could offer a PPO option in San Diego and Imperial counties. A selected group of participating providers in the San Diego/Imperial counties area could be organized as a network. A significant cost savings for the San Diego risk HMO might be elicited by establishing bundled pricing arrangements for services common to Medicare recipients, such as open heart surgery, hip replacement surgery, and oncology treatments.

One of the advantages of a PPO network option is the ability of enrollees to choose out-of-network providers, albeit paying a higher level of coinsurance or higher deductibles. Medicare beneficiaries residing in the Baja California area might be especially receptive to the U.S. PPO option. Many currently use the Mexican health care system for a majority of their care but prefer to cross the border for specialized services.

Medical Savings Account

With the passage of the Balanced Budget Act of 1997, Medicare recipients may choose the option of enrolling in a Medical Savings Account (MSA). Under this option, Medicare pays a premium for a high-deductible health insurance policy and deposits the difference between this premium and the Medicare capitation rate into the beneficiary's Medical Savings Account. Medicare beneficiaries in Northern Baja could use their savings accounts to pay providers in Mexico directly. Because care in Mexico is less expensive, it is likely that more Northern Baja residents would be able to cover all their costs with the funds provided and would not have to spend out-of-pocket. Also, if they did not use many services for several years, their savings accounts should be able to cover the deductible completely, as well as non-Medicare covered costs such as pharmaceuticals.

Other Options

Other alternatives include health care prepayment plans (HCPPs) and Competitive Medical Plans (CMPs). HCPPs form a cost contract between HCFA and a medical group to provide professional services. They are available to risk-averse companies and employer organizations may develop them exclusively for their members. HCPPs do not cover Part A institutional services. Similarly, HCFA regulations do not require CMPs to offer some basic services, including home health and mental health care. CMPs usually do not provide extra comprehensive services and may limit out-of-area coverage.

Developing an HMO Network for Northern Baja California

Bidding the Contract and Selecting Eligible Risk HMOs

HCFA or its representative could request competitive bids from San Diego risk HMOs, insurance companies, and nonprofit health plan providers interested in providing coverage to Baja residents. The application would include detailed information on how the HMO would administer the plan, ensure quality of care and beneficiary satisfaction, and ensure compliance among selected providers. In order to give Medicare beneficiaries in Northern Baja California a choice of plans and to create a competitive environment conducive to high standards, HCFA may want to select more than one HMO to develop plans during the first year. Although the San Diego risk HMOs would directly administer their networks and pay providers, HCFA could choose an administrative agent to deal with provider and consumer complaints and oversee enrollment procedures.

Developing the Rate Structure

The selected HMOs would then need to determine appropriate rates for Mexican providers. The adjusted average per capita cost (AAPCC) paid to risk HMOs represents an actuarial projection of what Medicare expenses would have been for a certain category of Medicare beneficiary had the person remained in traditional fee-for-service Medicare in a given county. The AAPCC is the basis of monthly capitated payments to HMOs under contract to HCFA. HCFA pays HMOs with Medicare risk contracts 95 percent of the AAPCC. The rate for the Northern Baja California HMO beneficiaries could be estimated by surveying the standard costs in the area and determining a trial rate subject to adjustment at the end of the year. It would include an estimate of services utilized in San Diego County and an estimate for services in Northern Baja California.

Plan Administration

Administration of the plan would be handled by the selected San Diego HMOs. Medicare-approved practices and charging mechanisms could be modified to apply to the providers on the Mexican side of the border. For example, the San Diego risk HMOs might contract with a Mexican subsidiary or insurer to pay claims, interact with providers, and provide quality assurance. The HMOs probably would need to formulate a modified coding of Medicare charges, perhaps reducing the quantity of coded diagnoses by 50 percent or more. They also would need to train providers on the rules, regulations, and objectives of the Mexican portion of the HMO and develop or purchase a current software package to track patient care.

Enrolling Beneficiaries

The enrollees would be Medicare-eligible residents from Northwestern Baja, an area extending from Tijuana in the north to Punta Banda in the south. Under current HCFA enrollment requirements, the HMO must have at least

5,000 enrollees and 75 Medicare enrollees. The more problematic requirement, however, is enrolling a population that includes no more than 50 percent Medicare and Medicaid beneficiaries. The administrators might need to develop a marketing plan that targets a diverse population in the region. Alternatively, the Northern Baja beneficiaries could be treated as residents of another county covered by an existing risk HMO in San Diego or Imperial counties. Currently, for instance, several Medicare risk HMOs in San Diego County also cover Imperial County.

The HMO network would enroll the Medicare beneficiaries on a first-come, first-served basis to the limit of its designated capacity and provide open enrollment periods of at least 30 consecutive days during each contract. Enrollees would be allowed to opt out with 30 days notice by written notification to HCFA.

Recruiting Providers

The San Diego risk HMO presumably would select providers based on their cost efficiency, medical reputation, and scope of services. The administrators would assure that potential providers can provide sufficient and appropriate care. As outlined in Chapter 6, a large group of providers currently exists in this area, and many providers expressed interest in serving Medicare beneficiaries. For example, the Family Care Clinic, one of the newest providers in the Rosarito area, has already implemented strict cost-effective practices, high educational standards for their physicians and staff, and a large array of specialized services.

Recruitment of providers would have to occur through personal contacts as well as mailings to the more prominent physicians of Northern Baja California. Providers could attend informational recruitment meetings discussing the main aspects of HMOs, capitation, and Medicare.

Centralized information on enrolled providers could be available through pertinent Internet sites and newspapers that reach the Medicare-eligible population in the Northern Baja California area. Newspapers that could disseminate this information include the *Baja Sun* and *South of the Border,* two Ensenada-based publications.

One concern is the lack of English-speaking physicians in the area. Although there is a group of physicians who speak excellent English, there may not be enough physicians or appropriate translators to handle a large increase of Medicare-eligible, primarily English-speaking patients.

Additional Administrative and Structural Issues

Regardless of the specific type of plan chosen, Medicare contractors involved in presenting a waiver application to HCFA would need to detail strategies to meet HCFA requirements for several important administrative and structural issues. The following section reviews challenges and recommends approaches to designing strategies within the Northern Baja California region.

Utilization Management

Utilization management programs to control utilization and cost of health services for the covered beneficiaries may serve as an obstacle to provider recruitment. Unlike indemnity plans where failure to comply with precertification programs increases the financial liability of the member, many HMOs impose a financial penalty for noncompliance on the provider. This could be a problem for providers in the Northern Baja California area who may not be as familiar with these types of managed care procedures. The contracting HMOs might want to address this issue through up-front training.

Quality Assurance

An internal grievance board could be established for the resolution of consumer issues, with one branch in Ensenada and one in San Diego. This might better facilitate problem-solving for consumers, since the two areas are culturally different and it would be more difficult to travel from Punta Banda to San Diego to register and discuss complaints.

In addition, a Medicare appeals procedure will need formulation in both Spanish and English, with the procedure carefully explained to Northern Baja California enrollees. HMO trainers or facilitators could be assigned to the Northern Baja providers for the first two years in order to assure enrollees' understanding of specific quality assurance procedures.

To ensure quality for the Northern Baja California area, HCFA or its contractees could contract with an entity that would serve as a Provider Review Organization in Baja. The California PRO could possibly contract with Mexican physicians and nurses to serve as peer reviewers. The acceptance concerning PRO procedures might be slow for providers in Northern Baja California, as service provision from this region has never included these types of detailed reviews.

As an alternative to the PRO, HCFA could contract with an independent entity to manage the quality assurance process. Whether HCFA or its contractees choose to form a PRO or to work through an independent entity, the San Diego risk HMO administering the program will need to be thoroughly knowledgeable about common practices and accepted medical procedures within the Baja area. An in-depth understanding of the Mexican system will allow the HMO and its contractees to offer appropriate solutions to unanticipated problems.

Technology and Telemedicine

The technology available to the Baja California providers is often not at the level encountered in the U.S. today and may pose a problem for the HMO. Individual doctors or even small hospitals may not have tens of thousands of dollars available to purchase needed equipment within a short span of time. In order for many clinics to be up to par with American standards, the HMO may have to invest money up-front for modernization.

Telemedicine would be an appropriate link between Mexican and U.S. physicians for consultations when necessary. Most hardware would need to be provided by the San Diego risk HMO, as many Mexican physicians do not have the available resources to purchase the necessary equipment.

Limitations

The limitations currently in force under HMO regulations would probably also apply to people enrolled in a cross-border plan. Experimental treatments available in Mexico but not allowed by the FDA, such as the medication Laetrile, could not be covered.

Malpractice Insurance

Whether or how U.S. malpractice laws would apply to Mexican providers or in cross-border situations is at present undetermined. If providers were required to carry malpractice insurance in Mexico at the level of providers in the United States, costs could become prohibitive. The United States HMO may need to underwrite part, or all, of this expense.

Turning Strategy into Action

The development of an HMO network to serve Medicare beneficiaries living in Northern Baja California could save HCFA money while providing valuable access to medical care for Medicare beneficiaries. Insurance companies, HMOs, and nonprofit health organizations have made remarkable strides in creating policies and programs to meet the needs of NAFTA-era border communities all along the U.S.-Mexico border. Although the structural and administrative issues are many, a market exists for a well-designed Medicare HMO in Ensenada, Rosarito, and Tijuana. The number of retired Americans and Medicare-eligible Mexican citizens will grow in the coming years, leaving more elderly who paid into the Medicare system without appropriate health care in their communities of residence. A partnership between HCFA, a respected San Diego risk HMO, and Mexican providers could fill both a market niche and provide basic human services to the retired communities of Northern Baja California.

Notes

1. Health Care Financing Administration (HCFA), *Health Maintenance Organization (HMO) 1997 Benefits Comparison–Southern California* (Washington, D.C., May 1997), n.p.

2. HCFA, *1998 Guide to Health Insurance for People with Medicare.* Online. Available: www.hcfa.gov/pubforms/98guide1.htm. Accessed: November 16, 1998.

3. Ibid.

4. Ibid.

5. Ibid.

6. Jeffrey John Stys, *Binational Collaboration in Health Insurance Services between the United States and Mexico: Issues and Innovations for the Texas Health Insurance Industry,* Special Project Report (Austin, Tex.: Lyndon B. Johnson School of Public Affairs, The University of Texas at Austin, 1996), pp. 32-34.

7. Missy Turner, "Aetna to Expand Cross-Border Health Plans," *San Antonio Business Journal,* (December 22, 1997), p. 2; and telephone interview by Ann Williams with Pablo Schneider, Consultant, Blue Cross/Blue Shield of Texas and Arizona, San Diego, California, April 1, 1998.

Part 4
Issues in Implementing Coverage

Chapter 10
Quality Assurance for Providers

by Susan Davenport

A N IMPORTANT COMPONENT OF EXTENDING MEDICARE BENEFITS TO MEXICO will be quality assurance issues related to the Mexican health care system, in particular those pertaining to medical personnel and hospitals. The Mexican health care system functions quite differently from that in the United States, and issues related to the credentialing of health care providers along with accreditation of hospitals and other medical institutions will need review. This chapter focuses on these issues, along with several related topics, in order to discuss options and ideas for ensuring the quality of medical care for Medicare beneficiaries in Mexico.

Physician Education and Credentialing

Education

Medical education in Mexico has several noticeable differences from that in the United States. Medical education in the United States typically begins after a student's completion of twelve years of elementary and secondary school and completion of a baccalaureate degree, which usually encompasses four years of undergraduate college education (a declining number of United States medical schools require only three years of college).[1] In Mexico, students are admitted after completing twelve total years of education, which encompasses a baccalaureate degree within the Mexican educational system.[2] Entrance examinations for medical school are somewhat similar; however, they are not mandatory in Mexico. In the United States a student is required to take the standardized Medical College Admission Test (MCAT), but in Mexico, admission examinations are specific to the institution and not all institutions require them.[3]

Once accepted in medical school, a U.S. medical student will begin four years of education, typically referred to as undergraduate medical education. The first two years are comprised of basic science studies with a minimal amount of clinical training during the second year. The students begin patient care during their third year of education, rotating through hospital-based clerkships in the basic specialties of internal medicine, obstetrics/gynecology, pediatrics, psychiatry, general surgery, and family practice.[4] In contrast, Mexican medical education consists of six years of education, divided rather evenly between formal teaching and clinical training, and the duration of supervised hands-on training is considerably shorter than in the United States. The initial seven semesters of undergraduate medical education in Mexico consist of formal teaching, including courses in the basic sciences, theory, general knowledge of contemporary medicine and application of medical principles, and an introduction to a variety of medical specialties. There is also an opportunity for the student to voluntarily obtain further formal education and training. Following four years of medical education, students serve in a pregraduate medical internship for one year in a hospital setting under the direct supervision of physicians. Finally, graduating medical students all serve a mandatory one-year term of social service, typically in rural clinics in underserved areas of the country. These clinics or facilities are responsible for the training and evaluation of the students.[5] This mandatory year of service will prove to be a significant factor in reciprocity issues discussed later in this chapter.

Differences in the medical education systems of the United States and Mexico are apparent in the areas compared above; however, some important components may be overlooked if one reviews only training requirements. According to a U.S. physician who was educated in Mexico, the philosophy of the educational processes are extremely different. He describes his education in a Mexican medical school as deeply rooted in philosophy and community care, with the focus of all education being on the successful entry into a community-based system of medicine. That differs, he believes, from the American system of medicine, which is heavily rooted in business.[6]

Licensing

The conferring of a medical license takes place after the successful completion of the basic medical education in both countries as outlined above, with the United States having an additional component. In the United States medical licenses are conferred by each individual state, with each state also having authority over professional regulation and public education. All states except one currently require a minimum of one year of Graduate Medical Education (GME) for licensure, and many require two or three.[7] (Graduate medical education will be discussed shortly in the context of credentialing.) Once a license is granted most, if not all, states require some form of continuing education prior to the renewal process.

Licensure for Mexican physicians is handled in a much different manner. Physicians can register to practice upon passing a university degree program and fulfilling the necessary obligations as an intern and the year of social service work. The medical diploma awarded by each university is endorsed by the Secretariat of Public Education through the General Directorship for the Professions. This office grants the physician a *Cédula,* a permanent license to practice medicine, which is valid nationally. Thus the formal system of licensing physicians is controlled by the Secretariat of Public Education and the schools of medicine. Graduates are required to register with the Secretariat of Health; however, beyond graduation from a medical school, there are no requirements to prove professional knowledge or competence once a general practitioner has obtained licensure. Unless the health authorities suspend the licensee for violating the law or not performing up to standards, the license is valid throughout the duration of a physician's professional practice.[8] Beginning in 1999 there will be a national exam that graduates of medical schools in Mexico will have to pass in order to obtain their licenses.

The most significant difference in the medical systems of these two countries lies in their credentialing processes. In the United States, the licensing and credentialing process of physicians actually begins during undergraduate medical education. During this period most U.S. medical schools require students to display a certain level of proficiency before systematically advancing during their education. This proficiency is demonstrated by taking Step 1 of the United States Medical Licensing Examination (USMLE), usually after the second year of study. Many schools also require students to take subject examinations of the National Board of Medical Examiners in one or more disciplines. In order to successfully complete undergraduate medical education in the United States, a student must pass Step 1 and Step 2 of the USMLE. Once a student has successfully completed these examinations, he or she is allowed to begin graduate medical education. As mentioned earlier, a physician is licensed by the individual state where he desires to practice, and almost all states require at least one year of graduate education prior to conferring a license. With this prerequisite, graduate medical education becomes a crucial part of the credentialing process, as well as licensure, in the United States. The total length of GME required for certification in a particular specialty ranges from three to seven years, depending on the specialty being pursued.

Certification

In the United States the role of certification is maintained by a private organization known as the American Board of Medical Specialties (ABMS). As of 1995, 24 medical specialty boards were approved by the ABMS and the American Medical Association.[9] These boards are responsible for maintaining standards and improving the quality of GME and physician care. In addition, they also collaborate with other agencies and organizations to determine standards and approve facilities and programs for specialty training. The boards evaluate the students in areas of academic preparation, skills, and experience and issue certification to those who successfully complete the training program and required examinations. These credentials are often required by certain physician groups or institutions in order to practice within their facilities or organizations. As mentioned above, most states now require at least one year of GME before they will issue a license to a physician. Physicians performing graduate medical education are issued a temporary license during their first year of residency, which is a limited license allowing them to practice with supervision. After their first year of GME is completed, they are eligible to take a state board examination and practice as a general practitioner. They often take the USMLE Step 3 at this point. This is common in the United States in order for residents to "moonlight" and earn extra income on their own time.

Mexico does have a system of certification boards, which are the equivalent of specialty boards in the United States, but they currently hold less authority by comparison. These boards are administered and overseen by a nongovernmental group known as *Consejos de Certificación de Especialidades Médicas* (Certification Boards for Medical Specialties). While these boards perform a valuable service, as in the United States, Mexican law does not prohibit general physicians from performing the duties of specialists. According to the Law of Professions in Mexico, physicians are only required to obtain authorization to practice in a specialty field from the Secretariat of Public Education following the completion of their medical education.[10] Basically, any physician can practice any specialty he desires, as long as the proper registration has taken place. In the United States, on the other hand, most reputable hospitals require that most physicians be board-certified or qualified in order to perform specific procedures.

In order to obtain true certification, a Mexican physician must first pass a national examination to enter into postgraduate training. Hospitals and universities authorized by the Secretariat of Health can then offer postgraduate training. Upon completion of the required training, students receive a diploma and the majority take an examination for board certification. At present there are 43 boards of specialists recognized by the National Academy of Medicine.[11] The boards are formed by their respective affiliated medical society and overseen by the *Academia Nacional de Medicina* (ANM, National Academy of Medicine) and the *Academia Mexicana de Cirugía* (AMC, Mexican Academy of Surgery). The academies act in an oversight capacity, focusing on standards for practice.[12]

In Mexico the examination for certification process covers both theoretical and practical aspects of the specialty. This examination is evaluated by a group of recognized physicians from different schools of training. There is also a recertification process in Mexico, which is often more complicated than the initial certification. The recertification process must take place after five years and before seven years have passed since the initial certification. This process is based on a professional merit system evaluated by each of the boards of specialists. As of September 1994, only 32 (74.4 percent) of the 43 specialty boards had established their recertification system.[13] However, it is important to note that many of the boards have not reached five years of existence yet and therefore cannot recertify their members at this time. In the 32 boards that have a recertification process, a total of 5,155 (14.8 percent) specialists have been recertified as of September 1994.[14]

In devising methods to ensure quality assurance for physicians in Mexico, the current system of certification will be important and warrants a more thorough analysis. A certified specialist in Mexico is considered to have the knowledge and skills necessary to practice as a physician in a medical specialty area. This ability must have been acquired through postgraduate studies in a recognized university or hospital. More and more physician organizations, group practices, and hospitals are requiring specialty certification before accepting physicians to practice. International Hospital Corporation currently requires all physicians practicing in their hospitals to have specialty certification, and many other hospitals are requiring the same.[15] The number of certified specialists rose from 22,399 to 34,787 between the years 1990 and 1994.[16]

The creation of a certification process in Mexico dates from 1972, when the National Academy of Medicine published a document called "The Development of Specialists and Regulations for Specialties" that constituted the basis for the present organization of the certification process.[17] The board of specialists that govern all specialty boards by the authority given to them from the National Academy of Medicine have the following basic objectives: (1) to control the level of academic preparation of the specialists; (2) to promote before hospitals and government authorities the regulations that establish the framework under which the specialists are allowed to provide medical services; and (3) to protect the interests of the certified specialists, and of the society which they serve, by providing assistance to hospitals and helping the general public to get medical attention from qualified specialists.[18] The board of specialists also provide quality assurance processes through the recertification procedures mentioned earlier in this chapter.

There are several specific requirements that the National Academy of Medicine mandates the boards of specialists follow: (1) the boards of specialists must be exclusively focused on evaluating the knowledge and skills necessary to perform a medical specialty, thus certifying those physicians who possess such qualities; (2) they must certify and recertify all those individuals who fulfill the requirements and voluntarily apply for certification; (3) the boards of specialists must be established in those areas of medical practice where there is a need to provide medical services; (4) the National Academy of Medicine must approve the creation of new boards of specialists; and (5) the boards must be comprised exclusively of physicians that belong to the specialty and that constitute a representative group from all over the country and from the various medical institutions.[19]

As mentioned above, specialty certification for physicians is gaining widespread support throughout Mexico. It will, however, logically take some time for integration throughout the country. What is important to our efforts are the current numbers of certified specialists in Mexico. To examine these figures, we can look at several pieces of information. First, the total number of licensed physicians in Mexico as of September 1994 was 173,926; 80.5 percent of these were active and 19.5 percent were inactive.[20] Of the active physicians, 21.1 percent are certified.[21] Out of 65,000 specialists in Mexico, 53.5 percent are certified and 46.5 percent are not certified in their specialty (as mentioned previously, the law does not require a physician to obtain certification to claim a medical specialty).[22]

In order to get a picture of Mexico's medical workforce we can look at a breakdown of where the physicians work. Of the total number of active physicians licensed in 1994, 43.2 percent of the physicians practiced in the social security institutions, 33.2 percent practiced in private institutions, and 23.6 percent practiced in public institutions.[23] We can also analyze the total number of physicians, board-certified physicians, and recertified physicians within each specialty board as of September 1994 from Table 10.1.[24]

As noted earlier, certification is becoming more recognized as desirable by Mexican physicians and the hospitals and institutions where they work. In providing alternatives for assuring the quality of medical care for Medicare beneficiaries in Mexico, we will undoubtedly look to some utilization of their current system.

Reciprocity Issues

It is worth mentioning here the reciprocity issues concerning physician practices between Mexico and the United States. At the present time, for a physician from Mexico to be licensed to practice in the United States, he or she must obtain certification from the Educational Commission for Foreign Medical Graduates (ECFMG) and complete Graduate Medical Education (GME) in the United States. Since licensure requirements in all U.S. states require at least one year of GME for International Medical Graduates (IMG) to be eligible for a new license, any physician from Mexico who wishes to be licensed in the United States will be mandated to perform additional training here.[25]

Table 10.1
Number of Board-Certified Physicians in Mexico by Specialty

Name of Board	Certified by 1990	Certified by Sept. 1994	Recertified by 1994
Consejo Mexicano de Certificación en Pediatría (Pediatrics)	3,628	5,993	245
Consejo Mexicano de Cirugía General (General Surgery)	2,691	3,739	440
Consejo Mexicano de Medicina Interna de México (Internal Medicine)	2,128	3,214	359
Consejo Mexicano de Ortopedia y Traumatología (Orthopedics and Traumatology)	1,945	2,762	22
Consejo Mexicano de Anestesiología (Anesthesiology)	1,718	2,397	378
Consejo Mexicano de Certificación en Medicina Familiar (Family Medicine)	372	1,234	
Consejo Mexicano de Ginecología y Obstetricia (Gynecology and Obstetrics)	731	1,216	271
Consejo Mexicano de Cardiología (Cardiology)	707	1,101	309
Consejo Mexicano de Oftalmología (Ophthalmology)	706	1,069	868
Consejo Mexicano de Radiología e Imagen (Radiology)	534	868	386
Consejo Mexicano de Cirugía Plástica, Estética y Reconstructiva (Plastic Surgery)	525	760	
Consejo Mexicano de Gastroenterología (Gastroenterology)	385	740	184
Consejo Mexicano de Otorrinolaringología y Cirugía de Cabeza y Cuello (Otorhinolaryngology and Head and Neck Surgery)	414	675	175
Consejo Mexicano de Psiquiatría (Psychiatry)	526	662	10
Consejo Mexicano de Médicos Anatomopatólogos (Anatomopathology)	484	577	60
Consejo Mexicano de Dermatología (Dermatology)	396	543	
Consejo Mexicano de Cirugía Pediatrica (Pediatric Surgery)	383	539	161

continued on next page—

Table 10.1 continued—

Name of Board	Certified by 1990	Certified by Sept. 1994	Recertified by 1994
Consejo Mexicano de Urología (Urology)	358	507	51
Consejo Mexicano de Medicina de Rehabilitación (Rehabilitation Medicine)	312	478	20
Consejo Mexicano de Medicina Legal y Forense (Legal Medicine)	46	430	
Consejo Mexicano de Certificación en Medicina del Trabajo (Labor Medicine)	313	425	
Consejo Mexicano de Neurología (Neurology)	276	399	51
Consejo Mexicano de Medicina Crítica y Terapia Intensiva (Intensive Care and Critical Medicine)	328	383	
Consejo Mexicano de Cirugía Neurológica (Neurological Surgery)	210	361	147
Consejo Nacional de Certificación en Infectología (Infectious Disease)	147	351	45
Consejo Mexicano de Neumología (Pulmonology)	360	345	179
Consejo Mexicano de Reumatología (Rheumatology)	246	319	115
Consejo Mexicano de Patología Clínica (Clinical Pathology)	222	316	104
Consejo Mexicano de Oncología (Oncology)	(started in 1992)	310	
Consejo Mexicano de Endocrinología (Endocrinology)	209	297	76
Consejo Mexicano de Hematología (Hematology)	195	269	117
Consejo Mexicano de Audiología, Foniatria y Comunicación Humana (Audiology, Phoniatrics, and Human Communication)	131	196	64
Consejo Mexicano de Angiología y Cirugía Vascular (Vascular Surgery)	136	167	75
Consejo Mexicano de Cirugía Maxilofacial (Maxillofacial Surgery)	(started in 1991)	167	
Consejo Mexicano de Nefrología (Nephrology)	75	155	

continued on next page—

Table 10.1 continued—

Name of Board	Certified by 1990	Certified by Sept. 1994	Recertified by 1994
Consejo Mexicano de Especialistas en Genética Humana (Genetics)	130	148	38
Consejo Nacional de Inmunología Clínica y Alergia (Clinical Immunology and Allergy)	70	119	67
Consejo Mexicano de Especialistas en Enfermedades del Colon y Recto (Rectal and Colon Diseases)	82	106	
Consejo Mexicano de Certificación en Radioterapia (Radiotherapy)	102	102	76
Consejo Mexicano de Geriatría (Geriatrics)	(started in 1992)	99	
Consejo Mexicano de Médicos Nucleares (Nuclear Medicine)	70	91	37
Consejo Nacional de Cirugía de Tórax (Thoracic Surgery)	73	86	7
Consejo Mexicano de Neurofisiología Clínica (Clinical Neurophysiology)	33	72	18

Source: Victor M. Espinosa de los Reyes, "La Evolución y el Estado Actual de la Certificación de los Especialistas en México" (Evolution and Current Status of Certification of Specialists in Mexico), *Gaceta Médica de México,* vol. 131, no. 1 (Jan.-Feb. 1995), pp. 79-80.

Only physicians from nations that have reciprocal agreements with Mexico are eligible to practice there after fulfilling specific criteria. Currently, Mexico does not have such an agreement with the United States. Basically, United States physicians are not eligible under the Mexican Constitution, which states, "the professional practice of foreigners will be subject to the reciprocity in the residence of the applicant."[26] For countries with such reciprocity agreements, the International Medical Graduate must obtain validation of his or her medical education from the SEP and present documentation of citizenship, a passing grade on professional examinations, a professional degree from the country of origin, study plans of the university attended, and proof of proper immigration status from the Ministry of the Interior.[27] After providing this information, the physician is still required to serve a six-month social service assignment in Mexico.

Nursing Education and Credentialing

Dr. William Nolen made the following statement in 1970: "No matter what size the hospital is, the people who run it are not the doctors, the administrators, or the members of the hospital board; hospitals are run by nurses."[28] In addition to physician quality of care in the Mexican system, the nursing care provided in Mexico will also be important to Medicare beneficiaries. Nursing education in the United States encompasses technical, undergraduate, and graduate-level instruction in the profession of nursing. Licensure is conferred by each state after successful completion of board examinations, which are specific to either vocational or registered nurse educational tracks. Each state has boards specific to both vocational nursing and registered nursing within the state, and these boards establish standards of practice and promulgate and regulate licensure laws. A brief review of the current educational and licensure tracks is appropriate in order to note the differences between the U.S. and Mexican systems.

First, the vocational nursing program is a clinically intensive one-year program that offers classroom instruction and clinical practice (direct patient care experience) in four basic areas: pediatric nursing, maternity nursing, geriatric nursing, and medical-surgical nursing.[29] This training is undertaken after a high school education or GED is obtained. Licensed vocational nurses (LVNs) work under the supervision of registered nurses in a technical, support-type manner. Upon successful completion of their year of study, they are eligible to sit for the licensed vocational nursing examination and be licensed within the state where they practice. Neither an LVN or a registered nurse (RN) may practice nursing in the United States without a valid license from the state in which he/she is employed.

There are three educational tracks a person may follow in order to become a registered nurse. Regardless of the track chosen, graduates of the three basic programs all sit for the same board examinations and are conferred with the same license. The purpose of the associate degree program is to prepare nurses to give direct nursing care in hospitals and other health care settings. Graduates possess technical nursing knowledge and skill with an understanding of the scientific principles of nursing care. The majority of these programs are located in junior or community colleges, with programs varying in length from two academic years to two calendar years.[30]

Approved three-year diploma programs are traditionally associated with hospitals. Graduates are prepared for nursing in acute, intermediate, long-term, and ambulatory care facilities. Diploma programs primarily focus on the nursing process as well as health restoration and management of patient care in clinical nursing areas in a hospital setting.[31] These programs typically encompass one year of basic academic course work followed by two years of nursing academic course work and clinical educational experiences.

Graduates of baccalaureate degree nursing programs are prepared to provide self-directed general nursing care and to assume leadership in planning, providing, and evaluating nursing care of individuals, families, and groups in a variety of settings. These programs stress health promotion including community health, health restoration, the nursing process, and management of health care in a variety of settings.[32] These programs are offered in university settings and encompass two years of basic, academic course work followed by two years of nursing academic studies and related clinical educational experiences. Upon completion of this program the student receives a Bachelor of Science degree in Nursing (BSN). In addition to undergraduate studies, universities offer advanced studies for nurses interested in master's and doctoral studies. These programs, along with advanced nurse practitioner programs (encompassing nurse practitioners, clinical nurse specialists, nurse anesthetists, and nurse midwives), prepare nurses for advanced nursing practice, leadership roles in administration and management, teaching, and research.[33]

One particular trend in nursing in the United States is worth noting. The nurse practitioner (NP) role, developed in the early 1970s in response to a shortage of primary care physicians such as pediatricians and family physicians, has grown substantially over the past 20 years and has demonstrated success and popularity.[34] NPs provide care to well and sick clients, usually in a clinic-type setting. They typically represent the "first line" of health care, especially in rural areas and for low-income families, emphasizing prevention of disease and injury as well as the identification and management of commonly occurring conditions such as infections, asthma, or minor injuries.[35] This specialized training is encompassed in specially designated master's degree programs.

The Mexican health care system currently supports three types of nursing roles. The first is the *Auxiliares,* or Auxillary Nurses, which constitute approximately half the current number of nurses in Mexico.[36] These nurses are trained in Auxillary schools that they attend after completing the equivalent of a high school education. There is no formal testing procedure upon completion of this program, therefore no license is conferred. There are currently no licensure laws concerning nursing in Mexico; nurses from all educational programs can perform the same duties and function in the same capacity.

The second type of nurses in Mexico are the *Técnicas,* or technicians, which are graduates of three-year nursing school programs.[37] These programs appear equivalent to the diploma programs in the United States. *Técnicas* are not baccalaureate graduates but do receive extensive education in nursing practice. There are numerous *Técnica* schools in Mexico.

The third category of nurses in Mexico are the *Licenciada en Enfermería,* or licensed nurses.[38] These nurses are conferred with a degree from a university and are given a license. There is no specific testing required to obtain this license, however, so it is honorary only. Nurses may enter this program after completing their high school educations, at which point the program will entail four years of study. They may also enter as *Técnicas* (having already completed three years of study) and complete a two-year course of further study in order to obtain their degrees and licenses. To have this degree and licensure in Mexico is still quite rare; however, the number of students is increasing. If a nurse in Mexico obtains a *Licenciada en Enfermería* she is eligible for graduate study or to pursue a master's degree.[39] At this final level a nurse will write a thesis, take specific examinations, and possibly sit for oral examinations. Upon successful completion of one or all of these components, the master's degree is conferred.

The descriptions of nursing education in Mexico seem to parallel those in the United States. The licensed vocational nurse of the United States appears similar to the *Auxiliares* in Mexico, although a greater portion of the Mexican nursing population are *Auxiliares* than LVNs in the United States. The associate degree and diploma nurses of the United States parallel the *Técnicas* in Mexico. The baccalaureate graduates in the U.S. seem equal to the *Licenciada en Enfermería*. With the absence of licensing by examination in Mexico, the differences in quality may be difficult to measure, though from an educational standpoint the programs seem similar.

The most significant difference between the United States and Mexico, other than the licensing issue, is in the actual practice of nursing. In the U.S., nurses are allowed to perform certain duties based on their educational training and license. For example, licensed vocational nurses perform a support role to the registered nurse and would not be allowed to perform certain procedures such as the administration of intravenous medications. Baccalaureate nurses are typically considered for managerial positions in the U.S. and many hospitals would require a BSN degree prior to the promotion of a nurse to such a position. In Mexico all nurses, regardless of their education or training, are allowed to perform any nursing-type function, and may do so in all clinical settings. There is no differentiation of tasks based on education, and with no licensing, distinguishing certain roles for specific types of nurses is impossible.

Hospital Credentialing

In the United States, most hospitals are credentialed by the Joint Commission of Accreditation of Healthcare Organizations (JCAHO). In Mexico, the situation is much different. Efforts have been underway for many years in Mexico to establish standards similar to JCAHO in the United States, but they have been unsuccessful to date. According to Dr. Enrique Ruelas, President and

CEO of Qualimed, S.A., in Mexico City, standards were close to being adopted around 1994; however, political changes took place at that time and the push for standards was abandoned.[40] Qualimed, an independent consulting organization, has made some strides in relation to hospital credentialing, but its approach is consumer-oriented and strictly voluntary in nature. According to Dr. Ruelas, up to ten hospitals in Mexico have undergone this voluntary certification, and the interest and demand are growing.[41] Qualimed, which Dr. Ruelas founded in 1995, holds as its mission the desire to contribute to the improvement of quality and efficiency of health care services through the setting and monitoring of quality standards, benchmarking information, clinical database design and analysis, training programs on quality improvement, and consulting. In 1984 Dr. Ruelas implemented the first continuous quality improvement program of any hospital in Latin America, involving physicians, nurses, and several other types of health care professionals, and since then has participated in consulting, teaching, and publishing. Dr. Ruelas worked on the voluntary hospital standards that came close to acceptance in Mexico in 1994. According to Dr. Ruelas, the standards were modeled after JCAHO regulations used in the United States and also standards currently in place within the Canadian system. Only minor changes were made to these models when formulating Mexican policies, mainly adjustments to account for cultural differences in Mexico.[42]

According to another source familiar with the health care arena in Mexico, the lack of consistent laws or regulations enforcing hospital credentialing in Mexico is frustrating. Public Health Law governs hospital entities; however, the observer has experienced different steps, rules, and regulations every time a new venture has been undertaken in Mexico. The reason for these discrepancies is that while the laws are federally mandated, enforcement is by state and local authorities. Any standards beyond the basic laws are voluntary in nature.[43]

The laws that apply to hospitals include a basic license requirement to operate the facility, which requires renewal each year. There are surprise inspections by state health inspectors; however, they look primarily for signs of gross problems, specifically sanitation aspects, and do not investigate hospital operations with any of the detail currently performed by JCAHO. There are certain regulations for specific hospital departments in Mexico, such as narcotics administration and radiation emission, which are reviewed by the state health inspectors, but once again they look for serious problems only.[44]

There is a report generated each year by the state health inspectors that identifies problem areas for hospital operation, but it does not report outcomes, morbidity and mortality numbers, or other measures. There is also a federal outcome document generated each year that provides statistics related to patient outcomes.[45]

Options for Ensuring Quality Assurance in Mexico

One possibility for assessing and confirming physician quality of care in Mexico centers around Mexico's current certification process for physicians, described in detail earlier in this chapter. HCFA could require all physicians treating Medicare beneficiaries to have certification from the *Consejos de Certificacion de Especialidades Medicas* (Certification Boards for Medical Specialties). Since these certifications are the closest to reciprocal standards currently in existence between the United States and Mexico, and a growing trend toward specialization in Mexico appears to be taking place, this option might be feasible. Physicians already practicing as specialists could either be required to obtain Mexican certification prior to treating Medicare beneficiaries or simply be grandfathered in.

Telemedicine could also play a role in assessing the quality of care provided by Mexican physicians. With the growing advances in this field it may be possible to have the care of Medicare beneficiaries coordinated by U.S. physicians through a telemedicine link with Mexican providers. A conference approach, so to speak, could allow the medical care decisions and applications to be discussed with a U.S. oversight physician. Reimbursement schedules for both the Mexican providers and the U.S. physicians could be negotiated to allow this conference approach to take place at the same cost of care as that provided in the United States. Follow-up concerning the care received would be important in assuring that recommendations have actually been implemented.

To ensure the quality of nursing care, one could maintain that since educational standards appear synonymous with the U.S. programs, nursing care should be considered synonymous. This would be somewhat tricky considering the lack of licensure and testing for nurses in the Mexican system. To require the *Licenciada en Enfermería* would be unrealistic due to the small numbers of graduates from these schools in Mexico to date. Since almost half of all nurses in Mexico are *Auxiliares* it would be necessary to place some restrictions on which type of nurses perform specific procedures. Since nursing service is typically a department of each hospital, the division of duties could be handled through specific policies and standards set up by the hospitals themselves. This would likely be the most effective route for maintaining high standards of nursing practice. Peer review and utilization review, as mentioned below, will also play a role with nursing care.

An important part of setting up quality assurance for service deliveries in Mexico could include some type of Peer Review Organization (PRO) such as those utilized in the United States. In addition, the basic practices of peer review and utilization review could be implemented with direction by HCFA. Another alternative would be utilizing hospitals in Mexico such as International Hospital Corporation, which already have stringent internal policies and procedures establishing a high quality of care. With their internal standards often taken from the JCAHO model itself, many of HCFA's concerns over quality of care might be alleviated by using these hospitals.

Finally, alternatives to assure quality of care in this region must be reasonable, well-planned, and carefully executed. We should expect a significant learning curve for the Mexican providers, as the entire arena of quality assurance is still new in most parts of Mexico. In addition, a sensitivity to the Mexican culture and current health care system will be paramount in gaining acceptance for these new ideas and practices.

Notes

1. David C. Warner, *NAFTA and Trade in Medical Services between the U.S. and Mexico,* U.S.-Mexican Policy Studies Program, policy report no. 7 (Austin, Tex.: Lyndon B. Johnson School of Public Affairs, The University of Texas at Austin, 1997), p. 126.

2. Ibid., pp. 127-128.

3. Ibid., pp. 126-128.

4. Ibid., p. 126.

5. Ibid., pp. 127-128.

6. Interview by Susan Davenport with Roy Reyna, M.D., Independent Consultant, Austin, Texas, February 18, 1998.

7. Warner, *NAFTA and Trade in Medical Services between the U.S. and Mexico,* p. 127.

8. Ibid., pp. 129-130.

9. Ibid., p. 127.

10. Ibid., p. 130.

11. Victor M. Espinosa de los Reyes, "La Evolución y el Estado Actual de la Certificación de los Especialistas en México" (Evolution and Current Status of Certification of Specialists in Mexico), *Gaceta Medica de Mexico,* vol. 131, no. 1 (Jan.-Feb. 1995), pp. 72-82.

12. Warner, *NAFTA and Trade in Medical Services between the U.S. and Mexico,* p. 130.

13. Espinosa de los Reyes, "La Evolución y el Estado Actual de la Certificación de los Especialistas en México," pp. 72-82.

14. Ibid.

15. Telephone interview by Susan Davenport with observer who wishes to remain anonymous, April 24, 1998.

16. Espinosa de los Reyes, "La Evolución y el Estado Actual de la Certificación de los Especialistas en México," pp. 72-82.

17. Ibid.

18. Ibid.

19. Ibid.

20. Ibid.

21. Ibid., p. 78.

22. Ibid.

23. Ibid., p. 77.

24. Ibid., p. 79.

25. Warner, *NAFTA and Trade in Medical Services between the U.S. and Mexico,* p. 131.

26. Ibid., p. 136.

27. Ibid.

28. Ruth Hansten and Marilynn Washburn, *I Light the Lamp* (Vancouver, Wash.: Applied Therapeutics, Inc., 1990) (brochure), n.p.

29. Board of Nurse Examiners, *Nursing Programs in Texas: A Fact Book* (Austin, Tex.: September 1992), p. 17.

30. Ibid., p. 23.

31. Ibid., p. 27.

32. Ibid., p. 29.

33. Ibid., p. 77.

34. Ibid., p. 87.

35. Ibid.

36. Telephone interview by Susan Davenport with Anna Marie Valle, Universidad Ibero Americana de Tijuana, Tijuana, Mexico, April 27, 1998.

37. Ibid.

38. Ibid.

39. Ibid.

40. Telephone interview by Susan Davenport with Enrique Ruelas, M.D., President and CEO, Qualimed, S.A., Mexico City, Mexico, May 6, 1998. Dr. Ruelas ob-

tained his medical education at the University La Salle in Mexico City and also holds a Master in Public Administration from the Center for Research and Education on Economics in Mexico City and a Master of Health Sciences–Health Administration from the University of Toronto in Canada.

41. Ibid.

42. Ibid.

43 Anonymous interviewee, April 24, 1998.

44. Ibid.

45. Ibid.

Chapter 11
Insurance Companies and Processes in the Mexican Insurance Market

by Horacio Aldrete and Ann Williams

THE INSURANCE INDUSTRY IN MEXICO REPRESENTED US$3.2 BILLION, OR 6.8 percent, of the total Mexican financial services market in 1995. The insurance services market contributed 1.4 percent to Mexico's Gross Domestic Product (GDP) and generated 19,398 jobs in Mexico in 1995. By comparison, the insurance market in the United States accounts for 8.53 percent of GDP, while in Canada and Japan it represents 6.46 percent and 12.64 percent, respectively.[1] According to the *Lagniappe Letter,* Manuel Aguilera of the Mexican National Insurance Commission predicts the insurance market will grow to represent 5 to 6 percent of GDP within the next 12 to 15 years.[2]

A September 1996 market report on the insurance industry divides the Mexican insurance market into three main groups: individual and group; accident and health; and property/casualty, which includes civil liability, marine/transport, fire, agriculture, credit, automobile, and miscellaneous. Of an estimated potential market of 10 million people, only 2.5 million have life insurance. Only 15 percent of the total housing market and one-quarter of the 11 million vehicles throughout the country are insured. During the first half of 1996, total sales of insurance premiums amounted to US$1.92 billion.[3]

Of the estimated US$3.68 billion insurance premiums sold in Mexico in 1996, health and life insurance represented 42.5 percent (38 percent for individual premiums and 62 percent for group plans) and property/casualty premiums accounted for the remaining 57.5 percent.[4] The total market in 1995 was estimated at $3.2 billion, with health insurance representing an estimated 9.5 percent, or approximately $304 million.[5] Other sources indicate that the Mexican Insurance Association estimated health insurance premiums at $320 million in 1996 and $420 million in 1997.[6]

Mexico has a total of 56 insurance companies that cover the market. The five largest insurance firms–Comercial América, Grupo Nacional Provincial,

Monterrey Aetna, Tepeyac, and Inbursa–account for 70 percent of the market. However, the participation of foreign investment in recent years as well as the expansion of the insurance market is expected to cause a decline in the market share of these top five companies.

Of the total premiums in 1995, 68.8 percent came from companies with local capital, 22.6 percent from firms with some foreign investment, and the remaining 8.6 percent from state companies. As of 1996, half of the 56 insurance companies in Mexico were financed with all local capital. Of the remaining firms with foreign capital, 13 were joint venture partnerships and 14 were subsidiaries of foreign companies.

The North American Free Trade Agreement (NAFTA) has enabled United States and Canadian insurance companies that had joint ventures in Mexico

Table 11.1
Insurance Firms with Foreign Capital Participation

Name	Foreign Investor	Origin	Percent Held
Aseguradora Inverlincoln	Lincoln Insurance	U.S.A.	49.0
Comercial América	Hicks Muse	U.S.A.	10.0
Chubb de Mexico	The Chubb Corp., Delaware	U.S.A.	9.27
	The Chubb Corp., New Jersey	U.S.A.	9.27
	Federal Insurance Co.	U.S.A.	9.27
Geo New York Life	New York Life	U.S.A.	35.0
Seguros Atlas	Republic Insurance	U.S.A.	30.0
Seguros Banamex	Aegon N.V.	Netherlands	40.0
Seguros Cigna	Cigna International Holdings	U.S.A.	49.0
Seguros Genesis	Santander	Spain	24.5
	Metropolitan Life	U.S.A.	9.99
	Metropolitan Tower	U.S.A.	7.91
	Metropolitan Asset Management	U.S.A.	7.2
Seguros Interacciones	Commercial Union	U.S.A.	44.0
Seguros Monterrey Aetna	Aetna International	U.S.A.	45.16
Seguros Tepeyac	Mapfre International	Spain	49.0
Seguros La Territorial	AGF International	France	32.46

Sources: U.S. Department of Commerce, U.S. Commercial Service, *Industry Sector Analysis: Insurance Services–Mexico,* Stat USA Market Report ISA960801, Doc ID 8777 (Washington, D.C., September 1996), pp. 1-37; and Comisión Nacional de Seguros y Fianzas, *Anuario Estadístico de Seguros 1997.* Online. Available: http://www.cnsf.gob.mx. Accessed: February 8, 1998.

Table 11.2
Insurance Subsidiaries with 100 Percent Foreign Capital

Name	Holding Firm	Origin
Allianz de Mexico	Allianz of America	Germany
Anglo Mexicana	Reunione Adriatica	Italy
Aseguradora Maya	American Bankers Insurance	U.S.A.
CICA, Seguros de Mexico	Combined Insurance Co.	U.S.A.
El Aguila	Windsor Insurance	U.S.A.
Gerling de Mexico	Gerling Konzern	Germany
ING Seguros	ING Northamerican Insurance	Netherlands
Liberty México	Liberty Mutual	U.S.A.
Pioneer	Pioneer Financial Services	U.S.A.
Principal International	Principal International	U.S.A.
Probursa	BBV	Spain
Seguros del Centro	GE Capital	U.S.A.
Seguros Colonial Penn	Colonial Penn (Lukadia)	U.S.A.
Seguros Interamericana	American International Reinsurance	U.S.A.
Seguros Renamex	Reliance Nation Insurance	U.S.A.
Skandia Vida	American Skandia Life	U.S.A.
Tokio Marine	Tokio Marine Delaware	Japan
Zurich, Cia. De Seguros	Zurmex Canada Holding	Switzerland
Zurich Vida	Zurmex Canada Holding	Switzerland

Sources: U.S. Department of Commerce, U.S. Commercial Service, *Industry Sector Analysis: Insurance Services–Mexico,* Stat USA Market Report ISA960801, Doc ID 8777 (Washington, D.C., September 1996), pp. 1-37; and Comisión Nacional de Seguros y Fianzas, *Anuario Estadístico de Seguros 1997.* Online: Available: http://www.cnsf.gob.mx. Accessed: February 8, 1998.

to increase their ownership share from 30 percent in 1994 to 51 percent in 1996. Foreign companies can increase their share to 100 percent in the year 2000. Between 1991 and 1995, 13 new foreign insurance affiliates were authorized to operate in Mexico. Seven insurance companies with foreign capital started operations in 1995: CICA, El Aguila, ING Seguros, Aseguradora Maya, Pioneer, Skandia Vida, and Zurich Vida. During the same period, four locally owned insurance companies obtained foreign capital participation: Atlas, Chubb, Monterrey Aetna, and Liberty.[7] Table 11.1 shows firms with foreign capital participation and Table 11.2 shows firms that are wholly owned by foreign interests.

The Health Insurance Market

Market Size and Growth

The Mexican private health care market, valued at over US$300 million, includes private employee group plans and individual health insurance. According to the United States Commercial Service, group plans accounted for $120.6 million of the overall market in 1996. The market for group plans was expected to grow by 10 percent, to $152.6 million, in 1997. For 1998 to 2000, the expected growth rate is 15 percent per year.[8]

Health insurance's share of total premiums more than doubled, from 4 percent to 9 percent, between 1988 and 1995. According to Seguros CIGNA, health insurance premiums grew 19.69 percent between 1994 and 1995, from $1.48 to $1.77 billion inflation-adjusted pesos.[9] Much of the growth is due to joint ventures between foreign and Mexican companies aimed at providing health insurance to employer groups. Other reasons for current and projected growth include the convenience and efficiency of private group health plans over traditional IMSS service and creation of new jobs due to the growth of the Mexican economy and NAFTA.

Approximately 36 companies offered medical insurance in 53 private hospitals in 1996. In 1995, Mexico's population of workers reached 33.9 million, or 36.8 percent of the total population of 92 million. Insurance business representatives estimate that 10 percent of the working population carries private health insurance coverage.[10] According to *Business Mexico,* Alfonso Castro, president of the Mexican Association of Insurance Agencies (AMIS), private group and individual plans supplement the primary care provided by IMSS. Castro predicts that the service packages currently run by hospitals and insurance companies will develop into organizations similar to HMOs in the U.S.[11]

Groups and Contracting

Insurance companies market major medical insurance to both employee groups and individuals. Insurance companies contract with hospitals to provide policies to employer groups at a 15 to 20 percent mark-up. The process begins with a firm requesting price quotes for a group plan from insurance companies. The firm seeking health coverage provides the following information: number of employees, risk associated with employees, and the extent of coverage sought. Once companies select a program for their employees, the employees choose from a list of hospitals in the insurance company's network. Group insurance policies last for one year.[12] Although employer groups often pay the total cost of the policy at the beginning of the year in order to negotiate lower rates, installment plans are available.[13]

Both hospitals and insurance companies marketing health services in Mexico often will work with small groups. One-third of Mexico's population is employed in approximately 1.3 million establishments, 97 percent of which are micro, small, and medium-sized firms.[14] Of Mexico's employers, 20,000 firms are defined as large, with more than 500 employees, while an additional 100,000 are medium, with more than 50 employees. Fewer than 50 employees each are employed by 1.18 million companies. The 120,000 large and medium firms accounted for nearly 90 percent of all medical insurance customers in 1997, and corporations hold 92 percent of all medical insurance policies.[15] With an annual budget of US$5.5 billion and 350,000 employees, IMSS serves approximately 35 million beneficiaries.[16]

Manufacturing companies, including food, metal products, and garment manufacturers, are the largest purchasers of private group plans, at 43 percent of total sales. Financial services companies and other service companies account for 32 percent and 21 percent of sales, respectively. The remaining 4 percent of sales are shared between individuals and firms in several other industries.

Mexican customers generally seek an annual medical insurance that gives them the opportunity to receive health care from a reputable hospital. They are also interested in using the hospital for primary care check-ups and in ensuring that coverage applies to family members as well.[17] HMOs as they are known in the United States are just beginning to appear in Mexico. As discussed in Chapter 9, Frontera Health Services began offering managed care in 1989 along the California-Mexico border. Currently, Aetna is offering a PPO in El Paso and cross-border HMO coverage with U.S. Healthcare, Seguros Monterrey Aetna, and Meximed on the California-Mexico border.[18]

MediPlan, a new and growing managed care organization in Guadalajara, offered one of the first managed care products in the interior of Mexico. A small group of Guadalajara doctors joined with Safe Passage International, a Denver-based brokerage firm, and Bienestar International, a health care company based in New York, to form the organization in 1996. Mediplan uses a managed-care system that employs primary care physicians and operates with a capitation system that pays physicians a fixed amount for each patient. As of November 1997, MediPlan had signed on 65 primary care physicians and 185 specialists and formed relationships with six hospitals and several clinics. The company is developing plans in seven other Mexican states. MediPlan hopes to offer individual plans by 1999.[19]

A joint venture between Mexican investors and Aaron Management has developed a network of franchised primary care clinics with headquarters in Chihuahua. The venture, called Family Care Clinics, currently has at least five clinics and plans to operate 100 clinics by 2000. Similarly, Grupo Angeles, the owner of a well-known hospital in Mexico City, plans to create an HMO to serve patients in a network of primary care facilities.[20]

The growth in private health insurance is putting pressure on Mexico's hospitals to grow and upgrade. Hospitals with 50 or more beds account for only 3.2 percent of the total number of private hospitals and are currently serving medium and large companies in Mexico.[21] According to the *Lagniappe Letter,* a 1994 United States Trade and Development Agency report stated that Mexico needs 30 new hospitals. The International Hospital Corporation, based in Dallas, completed construction of a new hospital in Hermosillo, Sonora, geared towards middle to upper-middle class Mexicans. The corporation recently opened a hospital in Chihuahua and plans to open a hospital in Puebla in 1999.[22] Current health care resources appear in the following tables: Table 11.3 shows private health care resources and Table 11.4 shows private medical facilities.

Regulation of the Insurance Market in Mexico

The Mexican insurance market is regulated by the *Comisión Nacional de Seguros y Fianzas* (CNSF) created in January 1990 as a decentralized agency of the Ministry of the Treasury. The CNSF supervises operations and ensures that insurance companies comply with the laws set by the Ministry of the Treasury. The legislative framework's authorization of the disclosure of financial statements and creation of investment regulations are among the most important functions of the CNSF. The basic laws that regulate all types of insurance in Mexico are the following:

- The *Ley Sobre el Contrato de Seguro* (insurance contract law) establishes the rights and obligations of the parties involved in an insurance contract.

Table 11.3
Private Health Care Resources and Locations in Mexico, 1994

	Medical Centers	Large Hospitals	Small Hospitals	Clinics	Total
Physicians	29,473	7,475	7,096	6,831	50,875
Anesthesiologists	3,143	755	605	474	4,977
Nurses	9,598	3,358	4,082	9,343	26,381
Hospital Beds	14,704	5,204	5,388	8,406	33,702
Outpatient/Emergency Beds	15,100	3,599	3,098	3,043	24,840
Inpatient Surgery Rooms	2,004	460	379	345	3,188
Outpatient Surgery Rooms	1,261	232	172	135	1,800

Source: U.S. Department of Commerce, U.S. Commercial Service, *Industry Sector Analysis: Insurance Services–Mexico,* Stat USA Market Report ISA960801, Doc ID 8777 (Washington, D.C., September 1996), pp. 1-37.

- The *Ley General de Instituciones y Sociedades Mutualistas de Seguros* (LGISM, general law of insurance companies and mutual societies) provides the legal framework for insurance companies concerning their organization, performance, accounting, inspection, and surveillance.

- The *Ley Federal de Instituciones de Fianzas* (LFIF, federal law of surety firms) provides the legal framework for surety firms.

- The *Reglamento de Agentes de Seguros y Fianzas* (insurance and surety agent regulation) regulates the scope and activities of insurance and surety agents.

The LGISM and the LFIF set the general principles, while the *Secretaría de Hacienda y Crédito Público* (SHCP, Ministry of the Treasury) and the *Comisión Nacional de Seguros y Fianzas* create and enforce the specific rules and requirements.[23]

Description of Selected Insurance Companies

Seguros Comercial América

Owners
Seguros Comercial América is owned by Grupo Pulsar Internacional, an industrial group founded by Alfonso Romo Garza in 1981. Grupo Pulsar Internacional has 25,000 employees and 66,000 commission-based sales rep-

	1-5 Beds	6-14 Beds	15-24 Beds	25-49 Beds	50+ Beds	Total Beds
State						
Baja California North	60	69	18	11	1	159
Baja California South	3	1	2	0	0	6
Jalisco	28	69	31	13	12	153
Querétaro	17	8	5	4	1	35
San Luis Potosí	7	11	5	2	2	27
Guanajuato	59	108	21	13	3	204
Mexico Total	**991**	**1,256**	**325**	**155**	**89**	**2,816**

Table 11.4
Private Medical Facilities in Selected States and Number of Beds, 1995

Source: U.S. Department of Commerce, U.S. Commercial Service, *Industry Sector Analysis: Insurance Services–Mexico,* Stat USA Market Report ISA960801, Doc ID 8777 (Washington, D.C., September 1996), pp. 1-37.

resentatives. Its business interests include insurance, financial services, construction systems, and agricultural biotechnology. In 1996 the industries that constitute Pulsar Internacional had global sales of more than US$2.5 billion.

Description and History of Company
Seguros Comercial América was created in 1993 as a result of a merger between Seguros La Comercial and Seguros América. These two companies were founded in the 1930s and were both leaders in the market even before the merger took place. In 1989, Grupo Pulsar Internacional acquired Seguros La Comercial and started to develop an aggressive expansion policy characterized by an enormous growth in the number of policies issued, net revenues, and technology development. In 1993, Pulsar increased its participation in the insurance market with the purchase of Seguros América. Despite the economic crisis of 1995, Seguros Comercial América continued its expansion policy and consolidated its leadership in the insurance market with the incorporation in 1996 of Aseguradora Mexicana (Asemex), a company formerly owned by the Mexican federal government. Beginning in 1997, Grupo Pulsar has planned to invest US$80 million to build 20 outpatient surgery centers in Mexico. With the acquisition of a 49 percent minority stake in Clínica Médica Sur (a major hospital in Mexico City), Pulsar took its second major step to offer health care services. Earlier in 1997, the company began building its first outpatient surgery center in Mexico City. Pulsar is targeting middle and upper class Mexicans who are more likely to travel to the United States for health care. The company believes that wealthy Mexicans would prefer to stay home if they could obtain high-quality health care in Mexico more easily.[24]

Location and Partnerships
Seguros Comercial América has more than 800 branch offices throughout Mexico and more than 11,000 authorized agents and administrative employees. The company also maintains two offices in the United States and has business relations with some of the most prestigious insurance firms in the world. The International Division of Seguros Comercial América provides services to multinational companies operating in Mexico and is in charge of the two international offices in Los Angeles and New York.[25]

Grupo Nacional Provincial

Owners
Grupo Nacional Provincial is owned by the Bailleres family. The Bailleres family has business interests in a variety of industrial and commercial firms and is considered one of the wealthiest families in Mexico.

Description and History of the Company

The history of Grupo Nacional Provincial goes back to 1901, when La Nacional Compañía de Seguros Sobre la Vida, S.A., was established as the first life insurance company in Mexico. In 1936, Seguros La Provincial, S.A., was founded as a property and casualty insurance carrier. These two companies were founded by Casa Woodrow, a broker for American and British insurance companies. In 1968 these two firms merged and formed what is now known as Grupo Nacional Provincial. At present, Grupo Nacional Provincial is one of the four largest insurance companies in Mexico and its assets reached approximately US$1.1 billion in 1995.[26] Grupo Nacional Provincial offers many types of insurance policies and controls almost half of the health insurance market in Mexico; its total sales for health insurance in 1996 were US$76,036,000, compared to US$84,298,750 for the rest of the market. In 1996, Grupo Nacional Provincial had 79,916 policies covering 185,548 beneficiaries, and paid US$45,228,283 in health benefits. In contrast, the rest of the health insurance market sold 95,801 policies covering 261,282 beneficiaries, and paid US$35,204,362 in benefits.[27]

Location and Partnerships

Grupo Nacional Provincial has its main offices in Mexico City and has branch offices throughout Mexico. The company offers a series of health insurance products called Línea Azul that allow the insured to visit doctors and hospitals in Mexico or in the United States.[28]

In October 1997, American General Corporation, a provider of retirement and life insurance services headquartered in Houston, acquired a 40 percent share of Grupo Nacional Provincial Pensiones, S.A. de C.V., a new holding company founded by Grupo Nacional Provincial. The holding company will own a 51 percent interest in Profuturo GNP, a company that provides enrollment, administration, and retirement services for employees with IMSS coverage. Profuturo GNP is the fourth-largest *AFORE* (*Administradora de Fondos de Retiro,* or Pension Funds Administration Company) in Mexico, with 1.2 million affiliates and a 12.8 percent market share. The holding company also owns a 100 percent interest in Porvenir GNP, a company that provides single-premium immediate annuities to individuals holding IMSS coverage.[29]

Seguros Monterrey Aetna

Owners

Seguros Monterrey Aetna is owned by Valores de Monterrey (51 percent of the stock) and by Aetna International. Valores de Monterrey is an industrial group that owns, among many other industries and businesses, Vitro (the largest glass production company in Mexico) and Bancomer (the second-largest financial group in Mexico).

Description and History of the Company

Seguros Monterrey Aetna is Mexico's third-largest insurance company. It leads the market in life insurance, maintains a strong position in the auto insurance market, and provides business insurance and employee benefits. Seguros Monterrey Aetna's direct sales force and brokers target customers from middle-income groups and small- to medium-sized firms. With more than 40 branch offices throughout Mexico, the company distributes its products through one of Mexico's largest insurance sales forces. Seguros Monterrey was founded in 1940 as a life insurance company; Aetna purchased part of the company in 1992, and from 1993 to 1996 increased its ownership to 49 percent of the company. As of December 1996, Seguros Monterrey had assets of US$921 million, revenues of US$556 million, and a work force of 3,000 employees and authorized agents.

Location and Partnerships

Through a partnership with Grupo Financiero Bancomer (GFB), Mexico's second-largest financial group, Aetna is a recognized leader in Mexico's financial services landscape. In 1996, Aetna and Bancomer formed a joint venture that will underwrite and distribute personal line products to Bancomer's customer base. Bancomer has the most extensive retail banking franchise in Mexico and operates 1,000 branch offices. The Bancomer/Aetna program will distribute life, auto, homeowners, accident, and health insurance. As a consequence of the recent privatization of Mexico's pension system, Aetna and its Chilean subsidiary, AFP Santa María, S.A., joined with Bancomer in another joint venture. The new pension administration company, Administradora de Fondos para el Retiro Bancomer, is becoming one of the largest in Latin America.[30]

Aetna has developed cross-border health coverage through Meximed, allowing members to receive health care coverage on both sides of the U.S.-Mexico border. These types of plans operate as a traditional health maintenance organization but use a network of physicians, hospitals, and health care services in Mexico.[31]

Seguros Tepeyac

Owners

Seguros Tepeyac is owned by Mapfre Internacional, S.A., Grupo Corporativo LML, and by José Luis Llamosas Portilla, who is also the company's CEO.

Description and History of the Company

Seguros Tepeyac was founded in 1944 and has become one of the most important insurance companies in Mexico. Seguros Tepeyac has a strong market share with more than 200,000 health insurance beneficiaries and also has strong positions in the auto insurance and life insurance markets. The company has more than 50 branch offices, 75 agencies, 800 employees, and 3,000 authorized agents throughout Mexico. More than 190 hospitals in Mexico and 5,000 hospitals throughout the world are eligible for coverage by the Tepeyac Health Insurance plan (including Methodist and United Health Care Hospitals). Tepeyac has developed customer-oriented products such as Meditel. This program, introduced in 1995, permits policyholders to telephone Tepeyac 24 hours a day and speak to a doctor regarding any medical problem or question, even if it is not an emergency. As one observer stated, "(t)he idea is to be as close as possible to the client so they feel protected by the company."[32]

Location and Partnerships

Seguros Tepeyac has more than 50 branch offices throughout Mexico and is a member of the MAPFRE System, the leading insurance group in Spain, with branch offices in 26 countries.[33]

General de Seguros, S.A.

Owners

General de Seguros is owned by a group of entrepreneurs including Arturo Ávila Novelo, John Luttman Fox, and Max Grunstein Tenenbaum. The company's chairman is Miguel S. Escobedo.

Description and History of the Company

General de Seguros was founded in February 1972 by a group of entrepreneurs with experience in the insurance market. Starting as a small company in Sonora, Mexico, General de Seguros has become one of the most important small to medium-sized insurance companies in Mexico. During the economic crisis of 1995 almost all sectors of the Mexican economy were affected by a market contraction, characterized by high interest rates (110 percent), high inflation rates (51.97 percent), and a devaluation of the peso of more than 100 percent. In this environment, all companies were pushed to decrease their fixed expenditures and to find new and better ways to stay in the market. Despite this adverse situation, in 1995 General de Seguros had profits of more than US$4 million and its total assets increased by 29.1 percent. The good financial situation of the company has enabled it to rapidly expand its operations throughout Mexico. General de Seguros provides many types of insurance policies and has a strong position in the health insurance market, where it offers an insurance plan called Salud Administrada (Administered Health) that has one of the most comprehensive benefits packages in the market.

Location and Partnerships
A totally Mexican-owned insurance company, General de Seguros, S.A., has its main office in Mexico City and has branch offices in more than 32 cities throughout Mexico.[34]

Seguros Inbursa

Owners
Carlos Slim Helú, one of the richest men in Mexico, owns Seguros Inbursa and the rest of the Inbursa Financial Group. A beneficiary of the privatization process in Mexico, Slim has interests in a wide variety of businesses and corporations. Perhaps his most remarkable success was the acquisition of Telmex, the national telephone company, which was practically a monopoly in the Mexican telecommunications market in the early 1990s.[35]

Description and History of the Company
The origin of Grupo Financiero Inbursa extends back to 1965. In 1984, Grupo Financiero Inbursa incorporated Seguros de Mexico, an insurance company founded in 1957 as Aseguradora Bancomer. During 1993, two more companies were added to this fast-growing financial group. These companies were Banco Inbursa (banking institution) and Arrendadora Inbursa (leasing firm). A year later, in 1994, Factoraje Inbursa (factoring firm) was created and incorporated to the group. In spite of the unfavorable economic conditions of 1995, Grupo Financiero Inbursa created two new firms, Operadora Inbursa de Sociedades de Inversión (mutual funds firm) and Servicios Administrativos Inbursa (administrative services firm). Seguros Inbursa is engaged in the provision of insurance policies and services for individuals and businesses. Coverage includes life, accident, health, automobile, and property and casualty insurance.[36]

Location and Partnerships
Seguros Inbursa maintains its main offices in Mexico City and has branch offices throughout Mexico. The company is currently considering the possibility of building hospitals for use by its 110,000 employees as well as other individuals.[37]

Challenges for Traditional Health Insurance Companies

Because health insurance does not comprise a large or important part of Mexican insurance companies' business, companies are only recently beginning to approach health insurance as a unique activity. For example, health accounts for only 8 percent of Comercial America's business. Less than 6 percent of the Mexican population has private health insurance. Most products are designed and marketed for upper-income groups who purchase private insurance as a supplement to IMSS. Furthermore, approximately 500,000 Mexicans travel to the United States for health care each year. Health insurers in Mexico will need to focus on recapturing this market.[38]

The large Mexican insurance companies offer a major medical product that often does not include primary care. Some companies tend to treat health insurance as a purely actuarial product much as they would a car or fire insurance plan. Mexican insurance companies contract with providers to offer specialty services and acute care on a fee-for-service basis. Because insurance companies reimburse providers at well below market rates, quality of care sometimes suffers. A physician who charges $50 for a procedure in Chihuahua, for example, can expect to receive $20 in reimbursement from Aetna. Although insurance contracts are usually set up so that the patient does not have to pay in advance and then request reimbursement, some providers who are tired of the slow payment practices of the insurance companies have begun to charge up-front.[39]

Plan Characteristics and Billing Procedures

Private health insurance plans cover from 70 to 90 percent of primary care costs, 100 percent of emergency care, and most surgery costs up to a limit that ranges from $20,000 to $100,000. Depending on the product, plans may cover additional services, including pharmacy, radiography, maternity, and optical care. None of the major companies have special plans for the elderly and some companies refuse to take patients over the age of 75. An exception is sometimes made for enrollees with 15 or more years of longevity in a plan.[40]

Enrollees usually choose from the insurance plan's list of providers and hospitals. In the case of planning a surgery, the patient seeks preapproval from the insurance company and works with a primary doctor. Although all the physicians involved in a surgery are paid separately (because they are not employees of specific hospitals but rather contract their services there), the primary doctor gathers information about charges from the surgeon, anesthesiologist, and other providers involved. The primary doctor then presents the charges in one bill to the patient's insurance company.[41]

The process of selecting and paying the hospital for various charges has been likened to purchasing services at a shopping mall with different vendors. Leticia Pérez Sanroman, Senior Trade Specialist at the U.S. Embassy in Mexico, uses a hotel analogy. Hospitals with fewer services can be likened to one-star hotels, while hospitals that offer the full range of services can be compared to four-star hotels. Services within hospitals are often separate businesses contracting with the hospital. Physicians, for example, usually own the radiology equipment. However, these sophisticated hospitals submit one bill to insurance companies and patients with a list of separate services. Some examples of line items on a bill include room charge per day, intensive care per hour, medicine and supplies, pharmacy, laboratory, and X-ray charges. Patients visiting smaller hospitals may have to find other providers to have X-rays and purchase prescription drugs. In the latter case, insurance companies require enrollees to submit an official prescription and original receipt. Primary doctors submit a patient history and explanation of need for the medication, X-rays, or laboratory services.[42]

Compliance and Quality Assurance

Insurance companies employ representatives called *asesores médicos* or *dictaminadores* to spot-check bills and procedures. Often, the auditors are trained physicians who, as employees of the insurance company, work with the administration of the hospitals to protect the interests of their companies. They function as caseworkers through the insurance plans' networks of hospitals for programmed and emergency care. Some challenges to the system include the lack of standardization of procedural coding and pricing (making it difficult to maintain systematic records that are comparable across providers) and that *asesores médicos* may be tempted to make deals with providers.

Systems and Automation

Mexican providers and health care companies use a variety of systems to automate patient records and billing procedures. The Family Care Clinics use a database developed in-house that employs CPT codes to track patient care. The company is currently working on the software to make it more similar to HMO software in the United States. Latino Health Services markets a Spanish-based software system that uses 380 CPT codes. MediPlan of Guadalajara currently uses the product and plans to further develop the system to use global identification codes in the near future. Two other, more developed systems in use include Erisco, a well-established client server with industrial capacity, and Diamond System, a system used by Meximed. Both systems have electronic verification software to determine plan eligibility.[43]

Case Studies of Private Medical Plans

Grupo Nacional Provincial's Línea Azul Internacional: A Case Study

Grupo Nacional Provincial offers a series of health insurance products called Línea Azul. Línea Azul Internacional allows the insured to visit doctors in Mexico or the United States. The network of covered providers includes hospitals in Mexico City and state, Guerrero, Hidalgo, Morelos, Querétaro, and Tlaxcala, as well as Arizona, California, Florida, Louisiana, and Texas.

In addition to coverage in network hospitals, the Línea Azul group of products provides members with access to Línea Azul Assistance. This assistance plan includes access to information about the policy and claims, medical consultations via telephone, and discounted medical fees with specialists, hospitals, laboratories, pharmacies, opticians, doctors' offices, orthopedic supplies, and rehabilitation and nursing services in the Línea Azul network.

Those insured with a Línea Azul product are also covered by an ambulance service in certain areas of the country called *Médica Móvil*. This service, also owned by GNP, provides for emergency care on board a mobile intensive care unit, emergency transportation for patients in critical condition, and home visits by medical personnel for nonemergency situations.

Línea Azul pays bills directly to providers within its network when surgery or treatment has been preplanned and approved. Physicians are required to file a medical report, bill for care at least five days before the procedure, and ensure that patients complete a form advising the company of details of upcoming treatment.

For emergency care that requires a hospital stay of more than 24 hours, the policyholder must obtain approval from Línea Azul via telephone from the hospital. Part of the approval process includes a visit from a company service advisor or *Asesor de Servicio* who explains the copayment and deductible process and delivers a summary of the visit costs at the end of the stay.

If the provider does not belong to the Línea Azul network, or if Línea Azul has not given preapproval, the policyholder must pay in advance and file for reimbursement. The process requires the policyholder to file original receipts, sickness and accident forms, medical and clinical reports, and a copy of the hospital file for the visit. Grupo Nacional Provincial analyzes the claim and determines whether and how much to reimburse the policyholder.[44]

General de Seguros' Managed Health Program: A Case Study

Description of the Program

General de Seguros, S.A., offers an insurance plan called *Salud Administrada* (managed health), which provides health insurance through three different plans: (1) Basic Plan, with maximum copayments, (2) Integral Plan, with minimum copayments, and (3) Total Plan, with no copayments. The health services covered in each of these plans are primary care, specialized care, dental care, maternity, hospitalization, and medicines. The managed health program also includes access to *INFOSAT,* a toll-free phone service that provides emergency medical assistance and customer services 24 hours a day.

In this program, the beneficiary selects a primary care physician from a network of affiliated physicians and specialists. The primary care physician is responsible for coordinating all aspects of the beneficiary's health care, including hospitals, laboratory services, pharmaceuticals, and referrals to specialists. In addition to coordinating the managed health program, the primary care physician has the following functions and responsibilities: ear and eye examinations, nonhospital services, authorization of ambulatory services, and authorization of emergency care. He or she also handles referrals to specialized physicians, pharmacies, diagnostic laboratories, and hospitalization services. As coordinator of the managed health program, the primary care physician verifies the eligibility of the patient, collects the copayment, and preapproves specialized care.

Compliance

The payment and compliance procedures vary slightly according to the different levels of medical attention. However, the managed health program coordinator uses five key elements in order to assure that services were provided. These elements are the identification card, the medical report, the dental report, the referral sheet, and the service order or prescription.

The beneficiary and his/her dependents are registered in the managed health program with an identification card. This identification card contains the personal information and type of coverage of the beneficiary. Services cannot be rendered without showing the identification card. The medical report contains the identification number of the patient, name and code of the physician, preliminary diagnosis, final diagnosis, Code of Therapeutic Procedures (CPT), International Code of Diseases (ICD), and the signatures of both the patient and the physician. The physician is responsible for filing this report. The dental report is filled out by the dentist and contains the identification number of the patient, name and code of the physician, a detailed description of the procedure practiced, the Code of Therapeutic Procedures (CPT), the International Code of Diseases (ICD), and the signatures of both the patient and the physician.

The primary care physician completes the referral sheet and submits it to the specialist who will provide the service. This form contains the identification number of the patient, name and code of the physician, previous diagnosis, specialist's diagnosis, and the CPT and ICD. Once the service has been provided, the specialist has to file a validation report and turn it in to the primary care physician, who will follow up on the procedure. The service order is used to refer the patient for laboratory testing or for prescription drugs. It contains the identification number of the patient and the name and code of the physician, as well as the description of the procedure performed or medicine prescribed.

After medical services have been rendered, the primary care practitioner gives the medical reports, referrals, and prescriptions to a *Coordinador Médico* (medical coordinator). The medical coordinator is a physician who works as a case manager and reviews the physician's diagnosis, the medical procedure, and the hospital and pharmaceutical expenses. Once the review process is completed and the medical coordinator has approved the claim, General de Seguros schedules its payment to the provider.

In some specific cases, a preauthorization process has to take place. This process is an approval by *Salud Administrada* of the services requested by the primary care physician before any medical attention is provided. The primary care physician has to obtain authorization from the Medical Director of Managed Health or from the Representative of Managed Health in the area to deliver the health services requested. Some of these special cases include hospital admissions, home nursing, ambulatory surgery (outpatient), rehabilitation services, MRIs (Magnetic Resonance Imaging), tomographies, and referrals in those cases where the patient has been referred to a specialist more than three times in a period of 60 days.[45]

The Role of IMSS Reforms

Special Clauses and New Regulations

The Mexican government passed legislation in 1996 that reformed the social security laws and widened the market for insurance companies offering private pensions and health insurance. Although the newly privatized pension system is already operational, the changes in policies regarding health policy have been slower to materialize.

Under current Mexican law, both employers and employees make mandatory contributions to the Mexican social security system (*Instituto Mexicano del Seguro Social,* or IMSS) to cover the cost of health insurance. Since 1943, Mexican law has included two clauses governing use of private health services. The new legislation and accompanying regulations provide guidelines to expand the clauses to a larger proportion of the population.

The first clause, *subrogación de servicios* (contracting of services), governs agreements with private health care service providers to provide health care to IMSS beneficiaries selecting that option. IMSS approves a third party to provide services and accept legal responsibility for IMSS beneficiaries. IMSS then pays the private provider a portion of the employer and employee contributions to cover the cost of the service.[46]

The second clause, *reversión de cuotas* (refund of contributions), allows companies to pay for private health coverage using their IMSS contributions. Previous policy allowed only banks and a few firms in Monterrey, who provided private health insurance to their employees before the advent of IMSS, to administer self-insured plans for employee health care. These companies currently receive 64 percent of employee and employer contributions in returned contributions. Approximately 30 companies and 250,000 employees are affected by these agreements.[47] IMSS would partially refund contributions paid for government coverage to enable companies to purchase the private plans.[48]

The new legislation allows IMSS to extend the *subrogación de servicios* and *reversión de cuotas* clauses to include additional beneficiaries, health care providers, and employer groups. The regulations will allow private providers to apply to be Private Health Administrators (APS) and contract with IMSS to provide services to beneficiaries. The expected new rules will allow a variety of companies to make agreements with unions or employers to contract with private providers for health care.[49]

According to an employee benefits survey by the insurance brokerage firm Brockman and Schuh, 91 percent of medium and large companies surveyed in Mexico already provide private major medical insurance to employees in addition to paying the IMSS contributions. Because IMSS has not allowed companies to substitute private policies for IMSS coverage and many employers regard IMSS coverage as insufficient, these companies make the decision to pay twice for employee health benefits.[50] Arturo Sanchez, an actuarial director with Alexander & Alexander, says that for smaller, less expensive services, people prefer to go to their private doctors, while they are forced to depend on IMSS for major medical treatment.[51]

Companies seeking to purchase private health insurance in place of IMSS have been required to provide a health policy that includes all of the benefits of IMSS coverage, including workers' compensation, unlimited coverage, and full service without a deductible.[52] The cost of this private health care as an employee benefit is deductible from corporate taxes.[53] Some companies offer private health insurance as an executive perk; however, it is only tax-deductible if offered to all employees. Mexican law makes any benefits mandatory after two years, so companies often avoid offering private health insurance as an official benefit.[54]

Regulations to accompany the law have been postponed several times. Sergio Torres, a partner with Brockman and Schuh, estimated in a 1996 interview with *Business Mexico* that the IMSS regulations would change within three years. At that time, IMSS was developing systems to allow companies to opt out of social security if individual employees agreed to the change.[55] An article appearing in the *Lagniappe Letter* in May 1997 still spoke in only general terms about the "promise of this liberated [health insurance] market" due to an overhaul in the social security system making "it much easier for employers to channel health care contributions to private insurers."[56]

Two articles in Mexico's *El Reforma* newspaper in March 1998 outlined governmental actions to implement the law and announced a completion date of June 1998 for the regulations. According to the article, in March 1999 between 8 and 15 percent (3 to 5.5 million) of IMSS beneficiaries will have the option to choose private health insurance over IMSS under the *subrogación de servicios* clause. Companies seeking to contract with IMSS to become Private Health Administrators will have six months to apply and demonstrate sufficient infrastructure. IMSS and governmental authorities will then have 60 days to approve or deny the application. Among others, Grupo Nacional Provincial, Seguros Comercial América, and Seguros Inbursa have been mentioned as interested in applying. Under the new regulations, the first beneficiaries who have chosen to "opt out" of IMSS would enroll in private plans beginning March 1, 1999.[57]

According to the *El Reforma* article, the success of the *subrogación* expansion will depend on the amount that IMSS decides to pay private clinics for providing health services. If those in charge of the regulations, which include IMSS, Banco de México, Secretaría de Hacienda y Crédito Público (Ministry of the Treasury), and the Secretary of Health, do not offer enough to attract providers, they may decide not to enter the market. Currently, 60 percent of employer and employee contributions is being considered, which is 4 percent less than banks receive under the *reversión de cuotas* clause.[58]

The Mexican government's reluctance to change the IMSS requirements stems from opposition from a variety of sources. The IMSS workers' union of over 300,000 opposes a larger role for private insurance companies in the provision of health services.[59] Although Gerardo Cajiga Estrada, the director of affiliation and coverage with IMSS, insists that the new regulations are not tantamount to privatization, some representatives in the Chamber of Deputies disagree. The Social Security Commission in the Chamber of Deputies argues that the government should be working to strengthen IMSS services, as opposed to replacing them. According to the *El Reforma* article, Gonzálo Rojas Arreola, president of the commission made up of the involved groups, suggests that the lack of appropriate equipment, infrastructure, and services in IMSS stems from a systematic drive to weaken the social security system in Mexico.[60]

IMSS Contributions

As of January 1997, required contributions changed from a flat rate to a variable rate. Employers, employees, and the government contribute differing amounts depending on the income of the employee.[61] The contribution rate for the government remains at 13.9 percent of the daily minimum wage. The employer's contribution rate was 13.9 percent in 1997, 14.55 percent in 1998, and will continue to increase at a rate of 0.65 per year to 20.4 percent in 2007. For employees making three times the minimum wage or more, the employer and the employee must contribute an additional payment that totaled 8 percent in 1997, 7.35 percent in 1998, and decreases each year by 0.65 to 1.5 percent in 2007. The employer pays about one-fourth of this sum and the employee pays the remaining three-fourths.[62] The average daily minimum wage in Mexico was N$24.40 (about US$3.05) in 1997, and N$28.08 (about US$3.51) in 1998.[63]

Mexican Insurance Companies as Medicare Intermediaries

The insurance market, private health insurance plans, and hospitals in Mexico have developed significantly during the 1990s. Both domestic and foreign companies continue to invest in health care infrastructure and private health insurance ventures. As evidenced by the section of this chapter providing case studies of two insurance companies, CPTs and auditing of services are accepted ways to charge, track, and confirm hospital procedures. Although fee schedules are not as involved as Medicare's RBRVS and DRGs and provider experience in administering private insurance does not compare to Medicare requirements, insurance companies have substantial administrative experience. Clearly, the Mexican health care system is prepared to tackle the training and retooling necessary to administer Medicare to eligible persons living in Mexico. The current market players and new entrants reviewed in this chapter have shown that they have the resources and technical experience that could potentially meet HCFA's requirements. In addition, they have the enormous competitive advantage of having ongoing relations with private physicians and hospitals throughout Mexico.

Notes

1.   U.S. Department of Commerce, U.S. Commercial Service, *Industry Sector Analysis: Insurance Services–Mexico,* Stat USA Market Report ISA960801, Doc ID 8777 (Washington, D.C., September 1996), pp. 1-37.

2.   Latin American Information Services, "Insurance Industry Report–NAFTA, New Reforms Promise to Advance Mexico's Faltering Market," *Lagniappe Letter,* vol. 13, no. 16 (August 2, 1996), p. 8.

3. U.S. Department of Commerce, *Industry Sector Analysis: Insurance Services–Mexico,* pp. 1-37.

4. Ibid.

5. Latin American Information Services, "Insurance Industry Report–NAFTA," p. 8.

6. Claire Poole, "Prescription Mexico," *U.S./Mexico Business,* vol. 4, no. 10 (April 1998), pp. 41-46.

7. U.S. Department of Commerce, *Industry Sector Analysis: Insurance Services–Mexico,* pp. 1-37.

8. U.S. Department of Commerce, U.S. Commercial Service, *Health Maintenance,* Stat USA Market Report ISA970301, Doc ID 7367 (Washington, D.C., March 1997), n.p.

9. Stephanie N. Ross, "Bright Future for Health Insurance," *Business Mexico,* vol. 6, no. 8 (published by the American Chamber of Commerce of Mexico, Mexico City, August 1, 1996), pp. 23-24.

10. U.S. Department of Commerce, *Health Maintenance,* n.p.

11. Oliver Libaw, "Long-Term Benefits," *Business Mexico,* vol. 7, no. 8 (August 1997), pp. 28-32.

12. U.S. Department of Commerce, *Health Maintenance,* n.p.

13. Interview by Ann Williams with Javier Flores, Market Research Specialist, United States Commercial Service, Mexico City, Mexico, March 27, 1998.

14. U.S. Department of Commerce, *Health Maintenance,* n.p.

15. Ibid.

16. Poole, "Prescription Mexico," pp. 41-46.

17. U.S. Department of Commerce, *Health Maintenance,* n.p.

18. Missy Turner, "Aetna to Expand Cross-Border Health Plans," *San Antonio Business Journal* (December 22, 1997), p. 2.

19. Robert Shephard, "First on the Scene: Mediplan," *Business Mexico,* vol. 7, no. 12 (Dec. 1, 1997), p. 64.

20. Latin American Information Services, "Social Security Reform Carves New Market for Private Investors," *Lagniappe Letter,* vol. 14, no. 10 (May 16, 1997), p. 10.

21. U.S. Department of Commerce, *Health Maintenance,* n.p.

22. Latin American Information Services, "Social Security Reform Carves New Market For Private Investors," p. 10.

23. Jeffrey John Stys, *Binational Collaboration in Health Insurance Services between the*

United States and Mexico: Issues and Innovations for the Texas Health Insurance Industry, Special Project Report (Austin, Tex.: Lyndon B. Johnson School of Public Affairs, The University of Texas at Austin, 1996), p. 18.

24. Denise Sicara, "Pulsar to Invest in Mexico's Health System," *The News,* Mexico City, Mexico (December 10, 1997) (Lexis-Nexis, n.p.).

25. Seguros Comercial América, *Nosotros,* http://www.segcoam.com.mx. Accessed: February 7, 1998 (Web site).

26. Grupo Nacional Provincial, *GNP: Coporativo,* http://www.gnp.com.mx. Accessed: February 7, 1998 (Web site).

27. Mexican Association of Insurance Institutions (AMIS), *Datos Estadísticos 1996.* Online. Available: http://www.amis.com.mx. Accessed: February 3, 1998.

28. Grupo Nacional Provincial, *Salud: Línea Azul,* http://www.gnp.com.mx/salud1.htm. Accessed: February 3, 1998 (Web site).

29. PR Newswire, "American General and Grupo Nacional Provincial Establish Strategic Venture" (Company News On-Call, press release dated October 2, 1997. Online. Available: http://www.prnewswire.com. Accessed: April 21, 1998.

30. Dow Jones News Retrieval, "Mexican AFORES Anticipate at Least Six Permit Awards," *Funds International,* Lafferty Publications Limited (January 1997), p. 11.

31. Turner, "Aetna to Expand Cross-Border Health Plans," p. 2.

32. Ross, "Bright Future for Health Insurance," pp. 23-24.

33. Seguros Tepeyac, *Inovación, Solidez y Liderazgo* (Innovation, Solidity, and Leadership), http://www.tepeyac.com.mx/tepeyac.html. Accessed: February 8, 1998 (Web site).

34. General de Seguros, S.A., *General de Seguros,* http://www.general-seguros.com.mx. Accessed: February 8, 1998 (Web site).

35. Geri Smith, "A Secretive Tycoon Gets Investor-Friendly: Carlos Slim Is Revealing Information about His Mexican Empire," *Business Week* (May 18, 1998), p. 166F.

36. Grupo Financiero Inbursa, *Historia,* http://www.inbursa.com.mx. Accessed: February 1, 1998 (Web site).

37. Poole, "Prescription Mexico," pp. 41-46.

38. Latin American Information Services, "Social Security Reform Carves New Market for Private Investors," p. 10.

39. Telephone interview by Ann Williams with Gustavo Novejas, General Director, Family Care Medical Systems, Chihuahua, Mexico, April 9, 1998.

40. Telephone interview by Ann Williams with Leticia Pérez Sanroman, Senior Trade Specialist, United States Embassy, Mexico City, Mexico, March 27, 1998.

41. Ibid.

42. Ibid.

43. Interview by Ann Williams with Pablo Schneider, Consultant, Blue Cross/Blue Shield of Texas and Arizona, San Diego, California, April 14, 1998.

44. Grupo Nacional Provincial, *Instructivo para el Pago de Reclamaciones* (*Línea Azul* Beneficiary Manual 1997-1998), Mexico City, Mexico, pp. 3-25 (pamphlet).

45. General de Seguros, *Salud Administrada 1997-1998* (booklet summarizing plan benefits), Mexico City, Mexico, n.p.

46. Jesus Castillo, "En Puerta, Privatización de IMSS," *Reforma* (March 10, 1988), p. 12A.

47. Castillo, "En Puerta, Privatización de IMSS," p. 12A.

48. Shephard, "First on the Scene: Mediplan," p. 64

49. Ibid.

50. Ibid.

51. Libaw, "Long-Term Benefits," pp. 28-32.

52. Ross, "Bright Future for Health Insurance," p. 23-24.

53. U.S. Department of Commerce, *Health Maintenance,* n.p.

54. Schneider interview.

55. U.S. Department of Commerce, *Health Maintenance,* n.p.

56. Latin American Information Services, "Social Security Reform Carves New Market for Private Investors," p. 10.

57. Jesus Castillo, "Afinan Privatizar Servicios del IMSS," *Reforma* (March 10, 1998), p.1.

58. Castillo, "En Puerta, Privatización de IMSS," p. 12A.

59. Latin American Information Services, "Social Security Reform Carves New Market for Private Investors," p. 10.

60. Castillo, "En Puerta, Privatización de IMSS," p. 12A.

61. Ross, "Bright Future for Health Insurance," pp. 23-24.

62. Secretaría de Salud (Ministry of Health), untitled printout containing schedule of payments, Mexico City, Mexico, 1996.

63. Secretaría del Trabajo y Previsión Social (Department of Labor), *Secretaría del Trabajo y Previsión Social,* http://www.stps.gob.mx. Accessed: March 1, 1998 (Web site).

Chapter 12
The Promise of Telemedicine

by Anjum Khurshid

N A RECENT REPORT BY THE INSTITUTE OF MEDICINE, TELEMEDICINE HAS BEEN defined as the use of electronic information and communications technologies to provide and support health care when distance separates the participants.[1] In the past few years, telemedicine has been increasingly used for delivering health services both within the United States and abroad. Studies have also shown that under certain conditions, the accuracy of diagnosis through telemedicine is almost the same as that in personal interactions between a physician and a patient. More and more physicians and patients are getting comfortable with the technology.[2] Telemedicine promises to revolutionize health care delivery mechanisms. The widespread use of the Internet and the World Wide Web has made the task of providing linkages much easier and more cost-effective than ever before. There is little doubt that telemedicine will become a significant mode of delivery of health services in the near future. The possibility of using telemedicine to provide coverage to Americans living abroad should be considered seriously by health professionals and policymakers.

When considering coverage of health care for Americans living abroad, telemedicine can play an important role in providing easy access to high quality health care. Many hospitals in the United States, such as the Mayo Clinic in Rochester, Minnesota, and Massachusetts General Hospital, are using telemedicine to provide follow-up services to their patients abroad. It is therefore quite possible for other medical facilities to extend similar services to their patients in Mexico. This chapter will discuss how telemedicine can be used to provide such services and what issues will be involved in such an arrangement. There will be a discussion of various telemedicine models that can be used for cross-border supply of services from the U.S. to Mexico. Since the existing telecommunications infrastructure determines what technology is feasible in different situations, a summary of the changes in the Mexican telecommunications industry as a result of NAFTA will be presented. Some ongoing projects using telecommunications in the field of health care will also be discussed. The chapter ends by examining the feasibility of using telemedicine for providing health coverage to Medicare beneficiaries in Mexico.

Transmission Technology for Telemedicine

Recent years have seen great advancements in telecommunications technology. These developments directly affect the options available for telemedicine programs. Several factors need to be taken into account when deciding on the type of technology to be used for these purposes. One of the most important determinants is the volume of data that needs to be transferred. The required speed of transfer of data is also important in deciding which technology to use. For live video and real-time links, high-speed connections are required, while for a store-and-forward process, the speed is not as important. The costs associated with establishing a telemedicine link are also vital in the choice of the transmission mode. The costs depend on the existing telecommunications infrastructure and the type of equipment on each end of the telemedicine connection.

In using telecommunications for health care, one needs to be able to transmit data accurately enough to serve the purpose of the link. The most basic form of telemedicine in use today is telephone conversation between a patient and a doctor or between two doctors. Telephone hotlines for dealing with emergencies, preliminary consultations for minor problems, and monitoring the status of patients at home are some examples of successful telephone use for health services in many countries. Plain Old Telephone System (POTS) is also the most cost-effective means of telemedicine. The downside to POTS is the severe limitation of data transfer in a medical consultation due to its low bandwidth.

The store-and-forward technique is the next advancement in technology that is used in telemedicine. Data sent from one site is downloaded at another site at a rate dependent on the bandwidth of the telecommunication link. If the amount of data transferred is large and the bandwidth of the connection is narrow, the transfer takes a much longer time. Conversely, with more bandwidth, even large amounts of data can be transmitted in a very short time. The most common use of the store-and-forward technology is e-mail. This is being successfully used to bring about appreciable improvements in sub-Saharan Africa and other parts of the world.[3] The M.D. Anderson Cancer Center in Houston is also using store-and-forward technology to provide follow-up services to its patients.[4] The advantage of this method is that it is far less expensive than any of the advanced technologies traditionally equated with the word "telemedicine." It does not contain live images or motion video, but it can serve a variety of purposes and bridge many gaps in health care delivery in underserved areas. Store-and-forward technology can be used for exchanging reports, opinions, images, and sounds. The ease and efficiency of using this technology combined with its low operating costs make it ideal for most telemedical work. People at either end of the link can work at their own convenience without having to schedule meetings. It also makes recordkeeping and archiving much easier.

Wavelet compression is a recent advancement in transmission technology that can transmit large amounts of data over existing bandwidths. This appreciably reduces the bandwidth requirement. Image compression or file compression, as it is called, allows the transfer of images over plain telephone lines because the image is compressed before transmission. The ideal for "lossless compression" (compression without any loss of image quality) is a 2:1 compression ratio, but the images are transmitted slowly in this case and require a very high bandwidth transmission line. While a JPEG (Joint Photographic Experts Group) compression yields 10:1 to 15:1 compression ratios, wavelet compression can cause compression of 30:1 to 50:1 with no visible loss of the image. It is so accurate that the FBI is using it to compress 30 million sets of fingerprints in its database for transmission to local law-enforcement agencies.[5]

The most advanced form of telemedicine is when live dynamic images and full-motion video is transmitted in real-time between two sites. It requires exorbitantly expensive equipment on both sides and also special communication links. Interactive full-motion video can be seen using broad bandwidth networks, including fiber optic cable and many satellite systems. The various wire services available for such transmission are T1 lines that have a capacity of 1.544 Mbits/sec, T3 lines that carry 44.736 Mbps/sec, and ATM (Asynchronous Transfer Mode) technology that carries up to 155 Mbits/sec. The ISDN (Integrated Services Digital Network) line, which uses existing telephone lines but different switches, is another service being widely used for transmission of data and video. However, there are difficulties in installation and in providing uniform access of ISDN even within the U.S. By using data-compression technology, interactive television may be used with somewhat narrower bandwidths (384 Kbps, or 1/4 T1) but the images transmitted by this method frequently appear jerky.[6]

Cost of Telemedicine Projects

The cost of any telemedicine project will depend on the equipment, transmission mode, technical advice, maintenance of equipment, training of personnel, and medical consultation fees. These are the broad categories that can be broken down into further detailed components. These categories will not have the same share of the total costs in all projects, however. The importance and cost of each component will vary with each project. Some of the variables that might affect the price are

- location (urban, rural);

- services to be delivered (imaging, monitoring, examination);

- purpose of the link (consultation, diagnosis, second opinion);

- existing infrastructure (telephone lines, fiber optic networks, satellite coverage);

Table 12.1 Description of Telemedicine Services	
Telemedicine Services	**Description**
Desktop telemedicine	Use of regular phone lines, ISDN lines, or cable to enable practitioners to interact with a remote patient, review medication, perform a visual examination, listen to the heart and lung sounds with an electronic stethoscope, and monitor vital signs
Electronic patient records	Used to keep patient records up to date and for the transmission of patient records, referral letters, and test results between general physicians and hospitals
Home health	Providing monitoring, advice, and regular visits through telecommunications
Medical emergencies	Telecommunications are being widely used to provide medical emergency services
Teleconsultation	Exchanging clinical information between physicians using telecommunications
Teledentistry	Video and telecommunications used for dental applications
Teledermatology	Deals with the skin and its diseases, mostly using transfer of images
Tele-education	The access to expertise and ongoing medical education of health care professionals and the public

continued on next page—

- frequency of use (emergency, daily, weekly); and

- workload (number of patients).

The Telemedicine Handbook, published in 1993, notes that the cost of starting up a simple telemedicine program in a rural hospital or clinic in Texas averages about $55,000. This includes $75 to $250 an hour for a telemedicine consulting team for assessment and design recommendations, $50,000 to

Table 12.1 continued—	
Telemedicine Services	**Description**
Telemetry	Provides a means for monitoring and studying human and animal physiological functions from a remote site
Teleophthalmology	Using telemedicine for diagnosing conditions related to the eye; involves transfer of data, images, and audio through videoconferencing, store-and-forward technology, or a combination of the two
Telepathology	Involves rendering diagnostic opinions on specimens at remote locations based on medical study of disease-related changes in cells and tissue
Telepharmacy	Telediagnosis by the doctor allows the doctor to send instructions to the pharmacist who supplies the medication to the patient
Telepsychiatry	Consultation where the psychiatrist assesses the patient by examination through a video link
Teleradiology	Electronic transmission of radiological images from one location to another for the purpose of interpretation or consultation
Telesurgery	Surgery at a distance using virtual reality concepts and robotics

Sources: William T. McCaughan, "Telecommunications Issues Impacting Rural Health Care in the United States and Texas," *Texas Journal of Rural Health,* vol. XIV (2nd quarter 1995), p. 6; Evan Rosen, "Personal Telemedicine; 1999: The Year of ADSL?" *Telemedicine Today,* vol. 6, issue 2 (April-May 1998), pp. 22-25; and Ace Allen and Terry Wheeler, "Telepsychiatry Background and Activity Survey," *Telemedicine Today,* vol. 6, issue 2 (April-May 1998), pp. 34-35.

$100,000 for purchasing equipment such as cameras and monitors, about $5,000 for installation, and $1,200 to $2,500 per month in transmission charges (on the lower range for a call-on-demand connection and a higher range for leasing a dedicated T1 line).[7]

Benefits of Telemedicine

Today, telemedicine is being used in almost every field of medicine. In many cases the use is limited to pilot projects, while in others it is well-recognized as an option for health services delivery. Teleradiology and telepathology are being increasingly used in hospitals in the United States as a means of reducing costs and increasing efficiency. According to an estimate, by early 1996 there were over 7,000 teleradiology units in the United States.[8] Similarly, home health is also employing telenursing stations to monitor patients at home.[9] Table 12.1 (pp. 200-201) gives a brief list of various telemedicine applications.

There are many proven and potential benefits of telemedicine. Some of the most obvious are improved access to care, reduced costs, reduced isolation, and improved quality of care. Improved access to care occurs due to greater health care availability in previously underserved areas, accelerated diagnosis and treatment, and a broader access to specialty care. Reduced costs are brought about due to decreased duplication of services, technologies, and specialists; increased availability of back-up services in general, or specifically during times of crisis; more effective distribution of resources; enhanced access to resources without necessity of travel; and opportunities for cost-effective relocation of medical service centers. Reduced isolation refers to professionals having more freedom in where to locate their practices, in that they can still obtain continuing education, specialty consultation, administrative support, collaboration, and peer support, even in rural areas.

Improved quality of care is brought about through enhanced decisionmaking through collaborative efforts (such as the referring physician, consulting physician, and patient working together simultaneously), greater continuity of care, centralized patient records, and opportunities to educate referring physicians so similar cases can be treated by that physician. Improved care also results from the greater patient involvement, knowledge, and compliance as the patient becomes an active part of the patient care team, and from the therapeutic sociological benefits seen as the family participates in consultations with the patient (for instance, in home health services through telemedicine, which may take place in the presence of family members).

Telecommunications Infrastructure in Mexico

The Mexican telecommunications infrastructure was underdeveloped until recently. The monopoly of the telecommunications industry by the state blocked the resolution of many of the impediments to development. Some of these problems included the following:

- outdated telephone lines and switching equipment that could not support many of the telemedicine applications reliably or quickly;

- tariffs and regulations within local service areas that greatly increase the cost of communication linkages;

- transmission charges, either dial-up or dedicated, that exceed the ability of the users to sustain the system; and

- potential inability of community facilities to absorb the fixed costs of telemedicine systems, such as equipment, maintenance, room modifications, utilities, support personnel and ongoing training, and hardware and software updates and modifications.[10]

Mexico's telecommunications industry is currently in a state of upheaval. Innovations are being introduced, modern technology is being adopted, and consumers are experiencing choices for the first time. The privatization process, which started almost seven years ago, has opened up the market to competition. The government realized that this is an industry that is susceptible to astronomical growth and to irreversible changes in short periods of time, and is therefore acting cautiously. It intends to stimulate the creation of new infrastructure and improvements in the quality of services, but does not want to lose control entirely to the highest bidder in the market. The key measures that have been carried out in this regard are opening long-distance telephone services, auctioning frequencies on the radioelectric spectrum, and auctioning the country's satellite system.

The Federal Telecommunications Law, passed in June 1995, is designed to provide mechanisms to grant concessions for telecommunications and satellite services. The law establishes the Federal Telecommunications Commission (*Cofetel*) to oversee this process of privatization and opening of the market. Specific concessions are required for companies that bid to exploit a public telecom network. Foreign companies are allowed to hold 49 percent of a concessions company and, with special permission, a higher percentage in the case of cellular companies. Long-distance concessions can be granted up to 30 years. They are renewable, require no fee to be paid to the government, and are awarded once certain simple requirements are met.

Long-Distance and Local Telephone Services

From 1991–one year after *Teléfonos de México* (Telmex) was privatized–to 1995, the telecommunications business, fueled by increased efficiency at Telmex as well as by new services, grew on average by more than seven times the rate of economic growth. During the company's first five years of private ownership, the number of working telephone lines increased from 5.2 to 8.9 million, and digitalization of local exchanges soared from 40 percent to almost 90 percent. Copper cables were ripped out of the ground to make way for a 30,000 kilometer fiber optic network that could carry more calls more efficiently and at lower cost.[11]

Nine long-distance concessions have been granted so far. Beginning January 1, 1997, competitors are now permitted to interconnect with Telmex's local network and gain access to ordinary telephones. The other main players in the industry include Aventel, Alestra, and Miditel. Avantel is a joint venture between Grupo Financiero Banamex-Accival (which owns Mexico's largest bank) and MCI. Alestra is a joint venture between AT&T, Telefonica Internacional of Spain, and Mexican conglomerates Grupo Alfa and Grupo Visa. It has completed a 4,600 kilometer multimillion-dollar fiber optic network.[12] Miditel is owned by a private Mexican interest (51 percent) and by Korea Telecom (49 percent), the telecom firm owned by the South Korean government. Miditel will work with STM Wireless, Inc., which earned a 10-year contract valued at more than $100 million, to provide and maintain a nationwide satellite network for telephone and data communication in Mexico. The satellite system STM provides makes it possible for users to call from any remote site to any other site within the network, eliminating the need for a central hub.[13]

By June 1997, according to figures from the *Cofetel,* which is overseeing the deregulatory process, 1.6 million users of Mexico City's 2.6 million phone service clients (60 percent) exercised their right to choose a long-distance company, and 53 percent of these selected Telmex. Alestra trailed in second place, with 26 percent. MCI's Avantel received 21 percent of the long-distance choices, while Iusatel won 0.22 percent, Protel 0.16 percent, Marcatel 0.10 percent, and Miditel 0.03 percent. Telephone customers who did not pick a long-distance carrier automatically remain with Telmex for a period of time.[14]

Radioelectric Spectrum

Wireless local loop services, which can lower installation costs for local telephone service by linking up remote areas with national networks through radio transmissions, have received special attention from the Mexican government. The government hopes that reduced costs will encourage competition with Telmex's local network. The government will auction concessions for 77 frequencies that can be used for local telephones. Except for cellular service, local telecommunications in Mexico until recently were the exclusive domain of Telmex. The Communications and Transport Secretariat expects radiowave frequencies, microwaves, and other wireless technologies to be the means for introducing competition in the local telephone market. Services included in the current auction for 20-year, renewable concessions are paging, UHF and VHF frequencies for private communications, wireless local access services, and two bands of personal communications services (PCS), which is an alternative to cellular service.

While long-distance carriers have been building their own cable-based networks, new providers of local service will use technologies such as fixed wireless communications, which are transmitted over radiowaves. Several companies already offer cellular service, though the market is dominated by Telcel, a subsidiary of Telmex. However, in June 1997, *Cofetel* announced that it had authorized a prelicensing agreement with Grupo Iusacell, under which a subsidiary of the cellular telecom company will provide local service on frequencies that were to be auctioned in October 1997. The move gave Iusacell a head start on its potential competitors, though it is reportedly limited to 50,000 subscribers.[15]

Satellite Services

Mexico's orbital satellites–*Morelos II* and the more modern *Solidaridad I* and *II*–are currently working at only 63 percent of capacity, providing satellite links for voice and data transmission as well as for television and radio. A fourth satellite, the state-of-the-art *Morelos III,* was to be launched in 1997. *Telecomunicaciones de México,* a state-owned company that currently operates the system, holds the rights for four more orbital slots for fixed services and is negotiating for acquisition of four additional slots for direct broadcasting services over Mexican territory.[16] The Mexican government decided that it will retain a 25 percent stake in the satellite concessions. It will sell off 75 percent of the shares in the system comprised of three satellites. Foreign investment will be capped at 49 percent and must take place as part of a venture with a Mexican company.[17]

Mexico's *Telefónica Autrey* and Loral Space & Communications of New York submitted the only offer in the Satmex (Satélites Mexicanos) auction in October 1997. Their joint venture was declared the winner of a 20-year, renewable concession and the two companies will pay about $688 million for the three satellites in operation, the rights to launch a replacement satellite, and ground operations. Loral, a major U.S. communications company, will expand into new markets with satellite services that include telephone transmission, high-speed data transmission, and broadcast technologies through public or private networks. Rural telephone service and data compression are some of the areas they hope to explore. In addition, the protocol signed on October 16, 1997, between the United States and Mexico will allow satellite operators on both sides of the border coverage of both countries and the ability to market their services to U.S. and Mexican customers. Loral plans to integrate the management and operations of Satmex into their Skynet operation, a data network they acquired from AT&T.[18]

Current Trends in Telemedicine in Mexico

Center for Distance Learning, University of Texas Health Sciences Center, San Antonio

The University of Texas Health Sciences Center (UTHSC) in San Antonio, Texas, arranges regularly to give lectures on various health topics through the UNAM (*Universidad Nacional Autónoma de México*) branch in San Antonio. In spring 1998, UTHSC offered a credit course in nuclear medicine to Mexican students at UNAM in Mexico City. UTHSC does not charge any additional fees for the course; Mexican students pay the normal tuition at their institution for the course.[19]

Universidad Nacional Autónoma de México Branch, San Antonio

The UNAM branch in San Antonio has a dedicated telephone line to the main campus of UNAM in Mexico City. They are the conduit for much of the videoconferencing between UNAM and U.S. institutions. Some of the activities that took place in 1998 are the following:

- a credit course on nuclear imaging by UTHSC during the spring 1998 semester;

- a series of monthly extended education dental programs, including lectures on AIDS in dental practices, by the UNAM dental school;

- a six-part series on medical trauma from Sharp Hospital, San Diego, and San Diego State University, in collaboration with UNAM San Antonio;

- a series of lectures by the South Texas Blood and Tissue Center on blood and tissue-related topics in collaboration with UNAM in San Antonio and UTHSC;

- an international interactive seminar in Spanish and French presented by

UNAM, the Franco-Mexican Association of Psychiatry and Mental Health, and the University of Paris; and

- a series of lecture programs on topics of technology innovation by the Southwest Research Institute in collaboration with UNAM San Antonio.[20]

There have been discussions about other programs for the future. There is a proposal to have regular "grand rounds" between UTHSC and UNAM. Methodist Healthcare Systems in San Antonio has shown interest in starting a link with UNAM in Mexico City. Also, Medical Destinations San Antonio, which promotes use of San Antonio health providers, had been involved in several lectures with UNAM in the past and is expected to develop some new initiatives using telecommunications.[21]

University of Texas at Brownsville

The University of Texas at Brownsville (UTB) has had close educational ties with the Technological Institute in Matamoros, Mexico, because of the geographical proximity of the two cities. The School of Medicine in Matamoros and UTB are considering the possibility of establishing a regular link through fiber optic lines between the two campuses. UTB has had frequent videoconference lectures through the UNAM connection in San Antonio. Currently, they usually use a microwave link for connections with Mexico; though not the most reliable, these are widely used because of the cost savings compared to T1 connections. According to Dr. Rene Sainz of Academic Computing at UTB, the infrastructure is well developed inside Mexico between most major cities. Mexico City and Matamoros are connected to cities like Guadalajara, San Miguel, and Tijuana through fiber optic lines. Therefore, the project at UTB would not only connect to Matamoros, but also to Monterrey, Guadalajara, León, and Mexico City via E1 lines (European standard, comparable to T1 lines in bandwidth).[22]

M.D. Anderson Cancer Center, Houston

The M.D. Anderson Cancer Center in Houston, Texas, is a superspecialty hospital reputed to be one of the leading centers in cancer research in the world. It has been using telemedicine for international and domestic consultation for several years. Videoconferencing is being used regularly with its branch sites in Orlando, Florida, and a clinic in Tyler, Texas. They also conduct multidisciplinary patient conferences for interactive treatment and treatment planning. They have held videoconference lectures through the branch campus of UNAM at San Antonio to establish links with the medical community in Mexico. Since most consultations are not of an emergency nature, the far less expensive store-and-forward technology can be used for transferring images between sites. The center negotiates its charges for consultations depending on the specific arrangements with different institutions. The factors considered include the load of cases, the requirements for direct or live consultations, and the training and education needs of the remote site.[23]

Telemedicine Center, Texas Medical Center, Houston

The Texas Childrens' Hospital is a part of the Texas Medical Center and is affiliated with the Baylor College of Medicine. It is one of the largest pediatric facilities in the U.S. The Telemedicine Center, though located in the Texas Childrens' Hospital, serves the entire medical center and also has a wide network of international telemedicine links. They have a regular association with King Faisal Hospital and Research Center in Riyadh, Saudi Arabia, and with Moscow in the field of cardiology. They have also had occasional links with the University of Malay in Malaysia, the University of New Queensland in Australia, the University of Vienna in Austria, and a university in Tel Aviv, Israel. The Telemedicine Center is playing an increasingly significant role in conducting grand rounds and interdisciplinary treatment conferences through telemedicine within the multispecialty Texas Medical Center.

The Telemedicine Center has also had previous contact with UNAM through the San Antonio branch by conducting a lecture through videoconferencing. The Telemedicine Center is interested in establishing contacts in Mexico, probably through contracts with health insurance companies in Mexico City. The charges for the services vary with the type of contract signed with the remote site. A comprehensive package including regular consultations, technical training, and exchange of fellows will have much higher costs than a link for second opinions where store-and-forward technology may be used and cases may be billed individually. The center is looking into state-of-the-art technology involving using the Internet for consultations between physicians and for patient "visits."[24]

Hughes Simulations International, Arlington

Hughes Simulations International in Arlington, Texas, is working with ISSSTE (*Instituto de Seguridad y Servicio Social para los Trabajadores del Estado,* or Social Services for State Workers) in developing a telehealth network in Mexico. It connects 16 cities all over the country through satellite connections of 512 Kbits per second. The cities connected so far include Tijuana, Chihuahua, Colima, Acapulco, and Mexico City. Ken Lucas, in the Virginia office of Hughes, also mentioned negotiations going on with IMSS (Mexican Institute of Social Security) to add telemedicine to their services. He was not aware of any direct telemedicine link between the U.S. and Mexico besides the UNAM branch in San Antonio.[25] The network in Mexico uses live videos, and the initial capital investment in the satellite technology often pays off in a year to

18 months, according to Ken Lucas. For instance, the results of a pilot project in telehealth by ISSSTE showed a 52 percent reduction in patient transfer with respect to the previous year. Hence, it is estimated by the project team at ISSSTE that even with a more conservative 30 percent reduction in patient transfer costs, the project pays for itself in two years.[26]

Medicare Reimbursement of Telemedicine

One of the most significant developments for telemedicine's future in the United States occurred with the passage of the Balanced Budget Act of 1997. Section 4206 of the act requires the secretary of health and human services to make Medicare Part B payments for professional consultation via telecommunications systems. It requires that the health care provider furnish a service for which Medicare would have normally paid and that the beneficiary reside in a rural county designated as a Health Professional Shortage Area (HPSA). In determining the amount of payment for telehealth services, the payments would be subject to Medicare coinsurance and deductible requirements, and balanced billing limits would apply to services furnished by nonparticipating physicians. Beneficiaries could not be billed for any telephone line charges or any facility fees. In addition, payment for telehealth services would be increased annually by the update factor for physicians' services under the fee schedule. The effective date for its implementation is January 1, 1999.[27]

The next section of the Balanced Budget Act states that the secretary of health and human services must conduct a four-year telemedicine demonstration project for beneficiaries with diabetes who reside in medically underserved rural and inner-city areas. The demonstration has several goals, including increasing access and compliance for chronic disease care and developing a model for cost-effective delivery in both managed care and fee-for-service applications. The telemedicine provider must be a "telemedicine network" defined as a consortium of at least one tertiary-care hospital, at least one medical school, no more than four facilities, and at least one regional telecommunications provider. The act also sets payments for services at 50 percent of reasonable costs. Costs include acquisition of equipment, curriculum development and training, telecommunication costs, and provider costs. There is a cap on payments of $30 million for the project.[28]

HCFA started a telemedicine reimbursement pilot project in October 1996 in four states. The project was intended to aid the agency in developing a reimbursement policy for Medicare. The four sites are West Virginia, North Carolina, Iowa, and Georgia. The three-year project is slated to end in September 1999. The demonstration involves for fee-for-service payments to a limited number of facilities in each state. Until recently, only three of the participating networks had submitted claims to HCFA for telemedicine reimbursement. The Medical College of Georgia, a 54-site network and the largest in the program, is still negotiating with HCFA on details at this writing. There has been a low utilization of claims as compared to the estimates of the agency. The agency had predicted several hundred claims during the first year of the project and an estimated expenditure of $111 million in telemedicine-related payments over the three-year time frame. Between January and December 1997, HCFA received only 60 to 80 claims from three participating networks. According to HCFA guidelines, consultant specialists receive the same pay for a teleconsult as for a face-to-face encounter. Primary care physicians work as telepresenters and receive only 50 percent of their usual reimbursement. The specialists receive between $70 and $140 per teleconsult while primary care physicians receive between $15 and $40.[29]

In the Medicaid program, any state may choose to reimburse providers for telemedicine services. Several states have implemented pilot projects of this kind. Currently, Medicaid programs in ten states cover some telemedicine services. These states are Arkansas, California, Georgia, New Mexico, North Dakota, Montana, South Dakota, Utah, Virginia, and West Virginia. Typically, the criteria that states consider before allowing telemedicine coverage is the availability of less-expensive alternative treatments, conformance with commonly accepted health care procedures, and the safety and effectiveness of the service. Radiology and interactive video consultations are some of the telemedical services often covered under Medicaid. The Montana Medicaid program, for example, supports telemedicine services to patients who are often more than 100 miles away from the nearest mental health or substance abuse practitioner. It was estimated that the use of telemedicine saved patients $65,000 in lost wages, food, and lodging in fiscal year 1995.[30]

Policy Issues Involved

Telemedicine may at first glance appear to be an activity mainly concerning technicians, electricians, and computer engineers, but the technological aspects are relatively minor compared to the policy issues associated with telemedicine. Telemedicine practice revolutionizes the whole concept of traditional health care delivery to an extent where new decisions and consensus have to be developed for aspects that have already been determined in the traditional health arena. Some of the issues that need to be addressed in any telemedicine activity between the U.S. and Mexico are briefly discussed below.

Liability
An important issue to be resolved in telemedicine is the issue of liability.

Medical liability laws may be somewhat similar in principle in Mexico and the U.S., but their application is a world apart. The U.S. system of health care has strict implementation of liability laws, and practicing medicine without adequate malpractice insurance is unthinkable for most physicians. In Mexico, however, the issue of liability does not hold any great importance in the practice of medicine. Most physicians do not have liability insurance against medical litigation.[31] This could be considered one less thing to worry about when establishing telemedicine links with Mexican hospitals. Currently, in most places in the world including many U.S. states, the doctor is considered to be transported to the location of the patient for the purpose of applicability of liability laws.[32] It is difficult to determine, however, if the extent of litigation and rewards of malpractice suits in the U.S. could influence more such suits to be filed in the U.S. by Mexican patients.

Costs

Despite recent advances in technology and the corresponding decrease in the cost of equipment, telemedicine may not be the cheapest way of delivering health care. But from a long-term point of view, telemedicine may still be a cost-effective way of providing high-quality health care to distant areas. Many Americans living abroad who return to the U.S. for health care spend a significant amount in travel costs and other associated expenditure. One of the main reasons for Americans voluntarily incurring this cost is their faith in the quality of health care in the U.S. With telemedicine links to U.S. hospitals, clinics and hospitals in Mexico can assure their patients a standard of care similar to what they expect in the U.S. Managed care has changed the way health spending and management is viewed in the U.S. Health insurance companies and organizations concentrate more on "whole health" and preventive medicine. In theory, a healthy patient in an HMO-type arrangement is beneficial for both the patient and the organization (an HMO or the government). Therefore, by keeping the American population healthy in Mexico, there will be cost savings for both the government in the case of Medicare recipients and to HMOs in the case of insured populations.

Reimbursement

In a study conducted by *Telemedicine Today* in conjunction with the Association of Telemedicine Service Providers (ATSP), of a total of 80 programs in 38 U.S. states, reimbursement was identified as the greatest barrier to program sustainability.[33] In Mexico this becomes an even bigger hurdle, with differences in currency and laws. There is such a difference in the living standards and incomes in each country that it will be difficult to compare rates for similar services in Mexico and the United States. As mentioned previously, with HCFA having to pay for telemedical consultations covered by Medicare in rural areas starting in January 1999, the process of establishing guidelines for reimbursement may be developed earlier than would be expected otherwise.[34]

Licensure

Physician licensure is an issue that can seriously undermine any efforts to establish viable telemedicine links with Mexico. As long as the consultation is between physicians on either side, the question of licensure would not be significant. But when the link is between a U.S. physician and a patient in Mexico, and reimbursement is added to the picture, the dynamics change appreciably. In the past several years Kansas, Nevada, California, Connecticut, Indiana, Oklahoma, South Dakota, Tennessee, and Texas have enacted regulations or legislation governing licensure of out-of-state telemedicine health professionals. Most states require physicians to obtain a full and unrestricted license in that state in order to offer medical services in the state. If Mexico follows suit on the basis of reciprocity, telemedicine consultations might be held to strict conditions of physician licensure.

Privacy/Security

Personal and privacy concerns are an aspect of new technology that is often underestimated as a determinant of success. With telemedicine consultations, patient records will be going from one country to another, and patients could feel they have no control over the flow of personal information. There is also the threat of unauthorized intrusion such as computer hackers who are able to tap illegally into private information on computer networks. It will be a challenge to overcome these fears and the technological difficulties to ensure privacy and security of information transmitted through telecommunications. The first step in this direction is to convince the physicians involved about the utility and safety of the system so that they can reassure their patients.

Interoperability

Differences in various systems of computers, telecommunications, and medical practice need to be reconciled to make successful connections between the U.S. and Mexico. For instance, Mexico uses the European standards for high-bandwidth lines, called E-lines, instead of the T-lines used in the U.S. The level of computer use in hospitals and doctors' offices is also much less in Mexico, hence further need for training and cooperation.

Language and Terminology

The language barrier may not have much significance, as many doctors in Mexico understand English and others would not mind learning it, as shown by their frequent attendance at seminars and training in the U.S. On the other hand, when dealing with patients who do not understand English, or with support staff who have problems communicating in English, telemedicine may encounter some serious barriers.

Telemedicine Project Possibilities

Telemedicine has shown itself to be technically feasible in many scenarios and to be cost-effective in the long run. It is also recognized to be one of the cheapest and quickest ways to improve access to health care in remote and rural areas. When looking at the use of telemedicine in the provision of health care to Social Security beneficiaries living in Mexico, various possibilities can be explored. Some of the different telemedicine projects that can be considered for the purpose of this study include patient monitoring, radiology and pathology diagnostic services, consultative services, educational services, and home health services.

Patient Monitoring

One of the most basic services that could be provided through telemedicine to Americans living in Mexico would be keeping track of patients of U.S. hospitals who are traveling or residing in Mexico. Since they are already under treatment in a U.S. hospital for which Medicare covers them, this might be a cost-saving process for the hospitals. It will also in all likelihood save Medicare by keeping their beneficiaries healthy while they are abroad, so they do not return sick and incur much larger expenditures in the United States. This is an effective way of establishing networks between institutions and countries. In any risk-HMO project in the Baja California area, establishing such networks for patient monitoring may also result in cost savings by limiting the number and kinds of services to be contracted in Mexico by the HMO.

Radiology and Pathology Diagnostic Services

If health care of American retirees is provided by an organization that has well-established links in the U.S., then they can use teleradiology and telepathology to get these services from these centers in the U.S. There would be no need to hire radiologists and pathologists in three different places. All that is needed is a remote transmitting site at the demonstration sites that can send their images to one place in the United States. In this case, the expenditures for these services would remain in Mexico for the most part. For example, the Arizona International Telemedicine Network performed the same laboratory services for several years using its facility in Tucson to provide results to Mexican hospitals. Using store-and-forward technology, the cost of sending images may become more feasible than employing a radiologist at each site of the demonstration project. It has the added benefit of controlling for quality more easily by having to monitor only one central hub site for required protocol and credentialing.

Consultative Services

More advanced links can also be established that would require a well-equipped clinic on the Mexican side. The initial cost of establishing such a clinic might be very high, though it may pay for itself over time if reimbursement policies change. With video and other diagnostic equipment, physicians in the United States could directly "see" patients in Mexico and get all the information they need through telestethoscopes and other such equipment. The physicians could hear the patient's heart and lung sounds, read their EKGs and EEGs, and talk to them face-to-face. All that is needed is a person functioning as a physician's assistant at the other end and an evacuation coverage for serious cases. M.D. Anderson Cancer Center charges between $100 to $250 for a store-and-forward consultation.[35] It might be much cheaper to cover such services through telemedicine than for the Medicare beneficiary to visit the hospital and possibly be kept for inpatient treatment at M.D. Anderson, at very high cost to HCFA.

Educational Services

One of the most fail-proof telemedicine links that can be established is that for training and education of Mexican physicians. With the wealth of knowledge available on the Internet through such reputable institutions as John Hopkins University, Baylor College of Medicine, and Stanford University, simple access to the World Wide Web could open up reams of information for practitioners in Mexico. They could benefit from details about various drugs, diseases, and procedures. They would also have ready access to the most recent literature in their respective fields of interest. If the need arises, special courses can be arranged as is being done by the UNAM branch in San Antonio.

Home Health Services

Home health is one of those telemedicine services that has proven to be cost-effective throughout the United States. Kaiser Permanente conducted a trial home health care project in Sacramento, California, where home health care nurses conducted video visits of their patients using telestethoscopes. Preliminary results showed that nurses can conduct about 15 visits per shift via video while they can make no more than six visits per shift in person.[36] Home health services that are covered by Part B can be provided through telemedicine from just one central location in each city. The central location can be staffed with a nurse or physician who is certified according to U.S. standards, so that the issue of quality is adequately addressed. With low-skilled help very cheap in Mexico, a video visit by a nurse from a central monitoring station can cut down on costs and at the same time ensure quality of care.

Conclusion

There are several different situations in which telemedicine may prove both a cost-effective and efficient means of delivering health care to Americans living in Mexico. However, while being technologically and financially feasible, other policy issues that have been discussed above might prove to be the biggest hurdles to overcome for its success. As shown by Mexico investing heavily in its telecommunications infrastructure and technological advancements driving the costs of equipment down, financing telemedicine projects would not be prohibitive compared to the savings and improvements that could be realized in health care.

Notes

1. Institute of Medicine (IOM), *Telemedicine: A Guide to Assessing Telecommunications in Health Care* (Washington, D.C.: National Academy Press, 1996), p. 36.

2. Mark Goldberg, Daniel Rosenthal, Felix Chew, Johan Blickman, Stephen Miller, and Peter Mueller, "New High Resolution Teleradiology System: Prospective Study of Diagnostic Accuracy in 685 Transmitted Clinical Cases," *Radiology,* vol. 186, no. 2 (February 1993), p. 429.

3. John Mullaney, *Thoughts,* http://www.healthnet.org/sn/sno496.html. Accessed: November 9, 1997 (SateLife website).

4. Interview by Anjum Khurshid with Lawrence Jones, Director of Telemedicine, M.D. Anderson Cancer Center, Houston, Texas, December 5, 1998.

5. Margaret Ryan, "Distance Health Care Is Latest Medicine," *Electronic Engineering Times* (April 29, 1996), p. 55.

6. Jim Grigsby, Margaret Kaehny, Elliot Sandberg, Robert Schleker, and Peter Shaughnessy, "Effects and Effectiveness of Telemedicine," *Health Care Financing Review,* vol. 17, no. 1 (Fall 1995), pp. 115-131.

7. Jane Preston, *The Telemedicine Handbook* (Austin, Tex: Telemedicine Interactive Consultative Services, Inc., 1993), pp. 34-36.

8. E.A. Franken, "Teleradiology Moving into the Mainstream," *Telemedicine Today,* vol. 4, no. 1 (Jan.-Feb. 1996), pp. 14, 25-26.

9. Evan Rosen, "Twenty Minutes in the Life of a Tele-Home Health Nurse," *Telemedicine Today,* vol. 5, no. 6 (December 1997), pp. 12-13.

10. Susan Stappenbeck, "The Potential Use of Telemedicine in the Delivery of Health Care between the United States and Mexico under NAFTA," unpublished paper written for a directed study supervised by David Warner, University of Texas School of Public Health, San Antonio, Texas, November 28, 1994, p. 12.

11. "Interview with Carlos Casasus, President, Federal Telecommunications Commission," *Latin Finance,* no. 85 (March 1997), p. M51.

12. Kevin G. Hall, "Long Distance Wars Begin in Mexico," *Journal of Commerce,* vol. 410, no. 28836 (October 24, 1997), p. 4A.

13. John O'Dell, "O.C.'s STM Inks Huge Mexican Wireless Deal," *Los Angeles Times,* Orange County edition, Business section (October 11, 1997), p. 1.

14. Jeff A. Wright, "Long-Distance Competition–Most Customers Choose Telmex," *The News,* Mexico City, Mexico (June 3, 1997) (Lexis-Nexis, n.p.).

15. Kevin G. Hall, "Mexico Decides to Limit Investment in Satellite System," *Journal of Commerce,* vol. 412, News section (June 17, 1997), p. 2A.

16. "Interview with Carlos Casasus, President, Federal Telecommunications Commission," p. M51.

17. Hall, "Mexico Decides to Limit Investment in Satellite System," p. 2A.

18. Mary Sutter, "U.S. Mexico Venture Mapping Plans for When It Takes Over Satellite," *Journal of Commerce,* October 31, 1997, World Trade section, p. 3A.

19. Telephone interview by Anjum Khurshid with Shaharzade Dowlatshahi, UNAM-USA Distance Learning and On-line Services, San Antonio, Texas, December 4, 1997.

20. Shaharzade Dowlatshahi, UNAM-USA Distance Learning and On-line Services, "Re: Delphi Study," Personal email to Anjum Khurshid, February 5, 1998.

21. Dowlatshahi interview.

22. Telephone interview by Anjum Khurshid with Rene Sainz, Educational Technologist Manager, Academic Computing, University of Texas at Brownsville, Brownsville, Texas, December 8, 1997.

23. Jones interview.

24. Interview by Anjum Khurshid with George Suhr, Texas Medical Center, Texas Children's Hospital, Houston, Texas, December 5, 1997.

25. Telephone interview by Anjum Khurshid with Ken Lucas, Hughes Simulations International, Arlington, Texas, November 2, 1997.

26. Javier Castellanos Coutina, ISSSTE, "Re: Delphi Study," Personal email to Anjum Khurshid, April 1, 1998.

27. U.S. Congress, *Balanced Budget and Reconciliation Act of 1997* (Washington, D.C.: Government Printing Office, 1997), sec. 4206.

28. Ibid., sec. 4207.

29. Kathy Kincade, "Low Payments, Red Tape Hinder Sites in HCFA Demo," *Telehealth Magazine,* vol. 4, no. 1 (February 1998). Online, n.p. Available: http://www.telemedmag.com/db_area/archives/1998/980201n1.htm. Accessed: March 7, 1998.

30. U.S. Department of Commerce, *Telemedicine Report to Congress* (Washington, D.C., January 31, 1997) (microfiche).

31. Class presentation by Pablo Schneider, Consultant, Blue Cross/Blue Shield of Texas and Arizona, Lyndon B. Johnson School of Public Affairs, Austin, Texas, October 21, 1997.

32. IOM, *Telemedicine: A Guide to Assessing Telecommunications in Health Care,* p. 33.

33. Bill Grigsby and Ace Allen, "4th Annual Telemedicine Program Review," *Telemedicine Today,* vol. 5, no. 4 (August 1997), p. 30.

34. U.S. Congress, *Balanced Budget and Reconciliation Act of 1997,* section 4206.

35. Jones interview.

36. Rosen, "Twenty Minutes in the Life of a Tele-Home Health Nurse," pp. 12-13.

Appendixes

Appendix A
Principal American Retirement Communities in Mexico

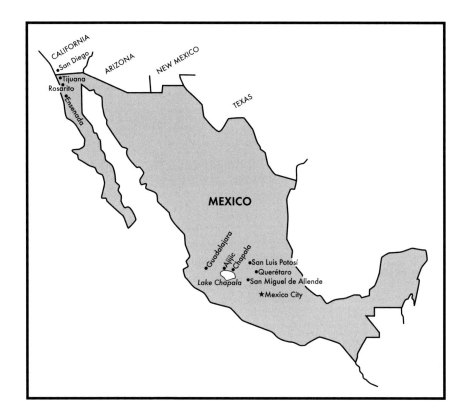

Appendix B
LBJ School Survey Distributed in Case Study Regions for Retirees Residing in Mexico

1. Do you currently receive:

Social Security Benefits	____Yes ____No
Veterans Administration Benefits	____Yes ____No
Civil Service Benefits	____Yes ____No
Military Retirement	____Yes ____No
Business Pension	____Yes ____No

Other (please specify)

2. Do you currently have an established source of medical care in Mexico?

____Yes ____No   In the U.S.? ____Yes ____No

Please specify established source in Mexico:

Name of Physician:

Facilities:

Locations:

3. In the event you needed to be hospitalized, where would you seek treatment?

Name of Hospital:

Address:

4. How do you pay for your medical care in Mexico?

     ____ Cash

     ____ IMSS

     ____ Private insurance (please specify carrier)

     ____ Other (please specify)

   How do you pay for your medical care in the U.S.?

     ____ Cash

     ____ CHAMPUS/Tricare

     ____ Medicare

     ____ Private Insurance (please specify carrier)

     ____ Other (please specify)

5. Do you receive home health care? ____Yes ____No

     If so, please specify the following:

         Average cost per visit:

         Services provided (medical treatment, cleaning, etc.):

         Reason for seeking home health care:

6. What was the total cost of medical care you have received in Mexico over the past three years? (specify amount in U.S. dollars, including amounts contributed by insurance benefits)

Cost of medical care received in the U.S.? (specify amount in U.S. dollars)

7. What was your personal contribution towards these amounts? (specify amount in U.S. dollars)

8. During the past three years, have you returned to the U.S. for health care services?

      ____ Yes ____ No

      If so, how many times?   Date of last visit?

      If so, why?

            ____ Lack of adequate medical care

            ____ More affordable medical care

            ____ Other (please specify)

9. What medical services were sought at that time?

      ____ Diagnostic   ____ Medical

      ____Routine medical examination   ____ Dental

      ____ Surgical (please specify)   ____ Emergency treat-
                                          ment (please specify)

      ____ Other (please specify)

10. In the event of a serious illness, do you feel that you would return to the U.S. for health care services?   ____ Yes ____ No

      If so, why?

      ____ Lack of medical services coverage

      ____ Lack of access to facilities or services

      ____ Inadequate local services

      ____ Other (please specify)

11. Have you purchased health insurance coverage in Mexico?

_____ Yes _____ No

Why or why not?

12. Have you bought into IMSS (the Mexican Social Security System)?

_____ Yes _____ No

13. If your Medicare or Veterans Medical Benefits could be used in Mexico, would you seek medical services there?   _____ Yes _____ No

If no, please explain.

14. If less than 65 years old, will you be eligible for Social Security in the United States?   _____ Yes _____ No

15. Additional Comments:

16. Date and Place of Birth:

17. Sex: _____ Male _____ Female

18. Marital Status: _____ Single   _____ Married

                          _____ Divorced   _____ Widowed

19. Number of members in household:

20. Occupation (if retired, please indicate previous occupation and how long retired):

How many years did you work in the United States?

21. Country of citizenship:

22. Are you a permanent resident of Mexico? ____ Yes ____ No

    If yes, how long?

    When did you last permanently reside in the U.S.?

    If no, please explain status:

23. What type of visa do you hold?

24. If you are not a permanent resident of Mexico, in which U.S. state do you hold permanent residency?

    Approximately how many months a year do you reside in Mexico?

25. In what city do you reside in Mexico?

____ Guadalajara	____ Lake Chapala
____ San Miguel Allende	____ Querétaro
____ Tijuana	____ Ensenada
____ Rosarito	____ Other (please specify community)

26. What is your primary reason for living in Mexico?

____ Cost of living	____ Climate
____ Family	____ Social
____ Business	____ Other (please specify)

27. Please indicate your current annual household income:

____ less than $15,000	____ $15,000-$25,000
____ $25,000-$35,000	____ Over $35,000

Appendix C
LBJ School Survey Results: Data by Question

This survey was conducted in late 1997 and early 1998 by the LBJ School graduate students researching each of the Mexican cities visited. Using the questionnaire in Appendix B, a total of 229 written responses were collected, including 85 in the Guadalajara area, 52 in the San Miguel de Allende area, and 92 in the Tijuana/Ensenada area. Retirees were located by visiting retiree organizations, handing out surveys in other locations frequented by U.S. retirees, and printing the survey in newsletters. Completed surveys were returned in person to the researchers while visiting in Mexico or by mail to the LBJ School of Public Affairs. We wish to emphasize that this is not a scientific survey and the data is for informational purposes only. The results are not statistically valid for all retirees as the respondents were not chosen randomly.

	Guadalajara		San Miguel		Tijuana/ Ensenada		Totals	
Question 1								
Social Security	85	(100%)	41	(78.8%)	67	(72.8%)	193	(84.3%)
Veterans Admin.	10	(11.8%)	4	(7.7%)	10	(10.9%)	24	(10.5%)
Civil Service	10	(11.8%)	2	(3.8%)	8	(8.7%)	20	(8.7%)
Military Retirement	1	(1.2%)	5	(9.6%)	3	(3.3%)	9	(3.9%)
Business Pension	18	(21.2%)	6	(11.5%)	23	(25%)	47	(20.5%)
Other	11	(12.9%)	10	(19.2%)	11	(12%)	32	(14%)
Question 2								
Mexican Source for Health Care:								
Yes	53	(62.4%)	19	(36.5%)	19	(20.7%)	91	(39.7%)
No	29	(34.1%)	28	(53.8%)	67	(72.8%)	124	(54.1%)
No Response	3	(3.5%)	5	(9.6%)	6	(6.5%)	14	(6.1%)
American Source for Health Care:								
Yes	45	(52.9%)	29	(55.8%)	66	(71.7%)	140	(61.1%)
No	25	(29.4%)	12	(23.1%)	14	(15.2%)	51	(22.3%)
No Response	15	(17.6%)	11	(21.2%)	12	(13%)	38	(16.6%)
Question 4								
Method of Payment in Mexico:								
Cash	71	(83.5%)	46	(88.5%)	67	(72.8%)	184	(80.3%)
IMSS	22	(25.9%)	2	(3.8%)	0	(0%)	24	(10.5%)
Private Insurance	9	(10.6%)	9	(17.3%)	9	(9.8%)	27	(11.8%)
Other	4	(4.7%)	2	(3.8%)	3	(3.3%)	9	(3.9%)
Method of Payment in United States:								
Cash	24	(28.2%)	8	(15.4%)	17	(18.5%)	49	(21.4%)
CHAMPUS/Tricare	1	(1.2%)	1	(1.9%)	0	(0.0%)	2	(0.9%)
Medicare	48	(56.5%)	32	(61.5%)	48	(52.2%)	128	(55.9%)
Private Insurance	27	(31.8%)	27	(51.9%)	42	(45.7%)	96	(41.9%)
Other	9	(10.6%)	4	(7.7%)	13	(14.1%)	26	(11.4%)

Getting What You Paid For

	Guadalajara		San Miguel		Tijuana/ Ensenada		Totals	
Question 5 Home Health Care:								
Yes	3	(3.5%)	0	(0%)	3	(3.3%)	5	(2.2%)
No	77	(90.6%)	52	(100%)	87	(94.6%)	216	(94.3%)
No Response	5	(5.9%)	0	(0%)	2	(2.2%)	7	(3.1%)
Question 8 Have Returned to U.S. for Care:								
Yes	24	(28.2%)	28	(53.8%)	66	(71.7%)	118	(51.5%)
No	57	(67.1%)	23	(44.2%)	25	(27.2%)	105	(45.9%)
No Response	4	(4.7%)	1	(1.9%)	1	(1.1%)	6	(2.6%)
Reason for Return:								
Lack of Care	0	(0%)	3	(5.8%)	6	(6.5%)	9	(3.9%)
Affordability	9	(10.6%)	10	(19.2%)	11	(12.0%)	30	(13.1%)
Other	13	(15.3%)	22	(42.3%)	36	(39.1%)	71	(31.0%)
Question 9 Services Sought in U.S.:								
Diagnostic	13	(15.3%)	17	(32.7%)	26	(28.3%)	56	(24.5%)
Medical	16	(18.8%)	9	(17.3%)	25	(27.2%)	50	(21.8%)
Routine	13	(15.3%)	20	(38.5%)	33	(35.9%)	66	(28.8%)
Dental	4	(4.7%)	7	(13.5%)	14	(15.2%)	25	(10.9%)
Surgical	6	(7.1%)	9	(17.3%)	14	(15.2%)	29	(12.7%)
Emergency	2	(2.4%)	2	(3.8%)	11	(12.0%)	15	(6.6%)
Other	2	(2.4%)	3	(5.8%)	7	(7.6%)	12	(5.2%)
Question 10 Would Return to U.S. for Care:								
Yes	41	(48.2%)	38	(73.1%)	74	(80.4%)	153	(66.8%)
No	27	(31.8%)	14	(26.9%)	16	(17.4%)	57	(24.9%)
No Response	17	(20.0%)	0	(0%)	2	(2.2%)	19	(8.3%)
Reason:								
Lack of coverage	21	(24.7%)	18	(34.6%)	33	(35.9%)	72	(31.4%)
Lack of access	7	(8.2%)	8	(15.4%)	9	(9.8%)	24	(10.5%)
Inadequate services	6	(7.1%)	9	(17.3%)	18	(19.6%)	33	(14.4%)
Other	30	(35.3%)	16	(30.8%)	24	(26.1%)	70	(30.6%)
Question 11 Purchased Mexican Health Insurance:								
Yes	31	(36.5%)	8	(15.4%)	5	(5.4%)	44	(19.2%)
No	53	(62.4%)	44	(84.6%)	86	(93.5%)	183	(79.9%)
No Response	1	(1.2%)	0	(0%)	1	(1.1%)	2	(0.9%)
Question 12 Purchased IMSS Coverage:								
Yes	33	(38.8%)	3	(5.8%)	0	(0%)	36	(15.7%)
No	52	(61.2%)	45	(86.5%)	90	(97.8%)	187	(81.7%)
No Response	0	(0%)	4	(7.7%)	2	(2.2%)	6	(2.6%)
Question 13 Would Use Medicare or VA in Mexico:								
Yes	81	(95.3%)	45	(86.5%)	71	(77.2%)	197	(86%)
No	3	(3.5%)	3	(5.8%)	11	(12%)	17	(7.4%)
No Response	1	(1.2%)	4	(7.7%)	10	(10.9%)	15	(6.6%)

	Guadalajara		San Miguel		Tijuana/ Ensenada		Totals	
Question 14								
Eligible For Social Security if Over 65:								
Yes	13	(15.3%)	10	(19.2%)	24	(26.1%)	47	(20.5%)
No	2	(2.4%)	4	(7.7%)	9	(9.8%)	15	(6.6%)
No Response	70	(82.4%)	38	(73.1%)	59	(64.1%)	167	(72.9%)
Question 16								
Where Born:								
United States	59	(69.4%)	43	(82.7%)	70	(76.1%)	172	(75.1%)
Mexico	2	(2.4%)	0	(0%)	0	(0%)	2	(0.9%)
Canada	2	(2.4%)	0	(0%)	1	(1.1%)	3	(1.3%)
Other Latin American	0	(0%)	0	(0%)	0	(0%)	0	(0%)
Europe	8	(9.4%)	1	(1.9%)	0	(0%)	9	(3.9%)
Other	2	(2.4%)	0	(0%)	0	(0%)	2	(0.9%)
Question 17								
Male	54	(64.7%)	29	(55.8%)	47	(51.1%)	130	(57.2%)
Female	31	(37.6%)	23	(44.2%)	43	(46.7%)	97	(42.8%)
No Response	0	(0%)	0	(0%)	2	(2.2%)	2	(0.9%)
Question 18								
Marital Status:								
Single	5	(5.9%)	7	(13.5%)	4	(4.3%)	16	(7.0%)
Married	48	(56.5%)	31	(59.6%)	55	(59.8%)	134	(58.5%)
Divorced	19	(22.4%)	7	(13.5%)	16	(17.4%)	42	(18.3%)
Widowed	12	(14.1%)	7	(13.5%)	13	(14.1%)	32	(14.0%)
No Response	1	(1.2%)	0	(0%)	4	(4.3%)	5	(2.2%)
Question 19								
Number in Household:								
One	34	(40%)	19	(36.5%)	24	(26.1%)	77	(56.8%)
Two	41	(48.2%)	27	(51.9%)	57	(62%)	125	(54.6%)
Three or more	6	(7.1%)	6	(11.5%)	7	(7.6%)	19	(8.3%)
No Response	4	(4.7%)	0	(0%)	4	(4.3%)	8	(3.5%)
Question 21								
Citizenship:								
U.S.A.	83	(97.6%)	50	(96.2%)	90	(97.8%)	223	(97.4%)
Mexico	1	(1.2%)	0	(0%)	0	(0%)	1	(0.4%)
England	0	(0%)	0	(0%)	0	(0%)	0	(0%)
Canada	2	(2.4%)	0	(0%)	0	(0%)	2	(0.9%)
Question 22								
Permanent Resident of Mexico:								
Yes	59	(69.4%)	35	(67.3%)	70	(76.1%)	164	(71.6%)
No	25	(29.4%)	17	(32.7%)	21	(22.8%)	63	(27.5%)
No Response	1	(1.2%)	0	(0%)	1	(1.1%)	2	(0.9%)
Question 23								
Type of Visa:								
FM-2	9	(10.6%)	0	(0%)	8	(8.7%)	17	(7.4%)
FM-3	59	(69.4%)	40	(76.9%)	53	(57.6%)	152	(66.4%)
Tourist	6	(7.1%)	6	(11.5%)	3	(3.3%)	15	(6.6%)

Getting What You Paid For

	Guadalajara		San Miguel		Tijuana/ Ensenada		Totals	
Question 25								
City of Residence:								
Guadalajara	23	(27.1%)	0	(0%)	0	(0%)	23	(10%)
Lake Chapala	47	(55.3%)	0	(0%)	0	(0%)	47	(20.5%)
San Miguel	0	(0%)	52	(100%)	0	(0%)	52	(22.7%)
Tijuana	0	(0%)	0	(0%)	3	(3.3%)	3	(1.3%)
Ensenada	0	(0%)	0	(0%)	34	(37%)	34	(14.8%)
Rosarito	0	(0%)	0	(0%)	52	(56.5%)	52	(22.7%)
Other	17	(20%)	0	(0%)	5	(5.4%)	22	(9.6%)
Question 26								
Reason for Living in Mexico:								
Cost of Living	57	(67.1%)	39	(75.0%)	68	(73.9%)	163	(71.2%)
Climate	66	(77.6%)	35	(67.3%)	59	(64.1%)	160	(69.9%)
Family	6	(7.1%)	2	(3.8%)	12	(13.0%)	20	(8.7%)
Social	20	(23.5%)	12	(23.1%)	30	(32.6%)	62	(27.1%)
Business	2	(2.4%)	0	(0%)	3	(3.3%)	5	(2.2%)
Other	8	(9.4%)	11	(21.2%)	17	(18.5%)	36	(15.7%)
Question 27								
Income:								
Less than $15,000	17	(20%)	10	(19.2%)	22	(23.9%)	49	(21.4%)
$15,000 to $25,000	30	(35.3%)	11	(12.9%)	19	(20.7%)	62	(27.1%)
$25,000 to $35,000	15	(17.6%)	14	(26.9%)	9	(9.8%)	38	(16.6%)
Over $35,000	19	(22.4%)	14	(26.9%)	34	(37%)	67	(29.3%)
No Response	4	(4.7%)	3	(5.8%)	8	(8.7%)	13	(5.7%)

Appendix D
LBJ School Survey Results: Selected Data by Location

San Miguel de Allende

	<$15,000		$15-25,000		$25-35,000		> $35,000		No Resp.	Totals
Household Size by Income										
One	6	(33.3%)	4	(22.2%)	6	(33.3%)	2	(11.1%)	0	18
Two	3	(11.5%)	7	(26.9%)	8	(30.8%)	8	(30.8%)	0	26
Three +	1	(16.7%)	0	(0%)	0	(0%)	4	(66.7%)	1	6
Have Mexican Insurance by Income										
Yes	2	(25%)	2	(25%)	2	(25%)	1	(12.5%)	1	8
No	8	(19%)	9	(21.4%)	12	(28.6%)	13	(31%)	0	42
Have IMSS by Income										
Yes	1	(33.3%)	1	(33.3%)	0	(0%)	0	(0%)	1	3
No	8	(18.6%)	8	(18.6%)	13	(30.2%)	14	(32.6%)	0	43

Guadalajara

	<$15,000		$15-25,000		$25-35,000		> $35,000		No Resp.	Totals
Household Size by Income										
One	10	(29.4%)	16	(47.1%)	4	(11.8%)	3	(8.8%)	1	34
Two	3	(7.1%)	11	(26.2%)	10	(23.8%)	15	(35.7%)	3	42
Three +	1	(14.3%)	5	(71.4%)	0	(0%)	1	(14.3%)	0	7
Have Mexican Insurance by Income										
Yes	7	(22.6%)	14	(45.2%)	3	(9.7%)	6	(19.4%)	1	31
No	10	(18.2%)	18	(32.7%)	11	(20%)	13	(23.6%)	3	55
Have IMSS by Income										
Yes	10	(30.3%)	12	(36.4%)	3	(9.1%)	6	(18.2%)	2	33
No	7	(13%)	20	(37%)	12	(22.2%)	13	(24.1%)	2	54

Tijuana

	<$15,000		$15-25,000		$25-35,000		> $35,000		No Resp.	Totals
Household Size by Income										
One	8	(33.3%)	10	(41.7%)	1	(4.2%)	3	(12.5%)	2	24
Two	10	(17.5%)	9	(15.8%)	5	(8.8%)	28	(49.1%)	5	57
Three +	2	(28.6%)	0	(0%)	2	(28.6%)	3	(42.9%)	0	7
Have Mexican Insurance by Income										
Yes	0	(0%)	1	(50%)	0	(0%)	2	(100%)	2	5
No	22	(25.6%)	18	(20.9%)	9	(10.5%)	32	(37.2%)	5	86
Have IMSS by Income										
Yes	0	(0%)	0	(0%)	0	(0%)	0	(0%)	0	0
No	21	(23.3%)	19	(21.1%)	9	(10%)	34	(37.8%)	7	90

Getting What You Paid For

Aggregates

	<$15,000		$15-25,000		$25-35,000		> $35,000		No Resp.	Totals
Household Size by Income										
One	24	(31.6%)	30	(39.5%)	11	(14.5%)	8	(10.5%)	3	76
Two	16	(12.8%)	27	(21.6%)	23	(18.4%)	51	(40.8%)	8	125
Three +	4	(20.0%)	5	(25.0%)	2	(10%)	8	(40%)	1	20
Have Mexican Insurance by Income										
Yes	9	(20%)	17	(37.8%)	5	(11.1%)	9	(20%)	5	45
No	40	(21.9%)	45	(24.6%)	32	(17.5%)	58	(31.7%)	8	183
Have IMSS by Income										
Yes	11	(30.6%)	13	(36.1%)	3	(8.3%)	6	(16.7%)	3	36
No	36	(19.3%)	47	(25.1%)	34	(18.2%)	61	(32.6%)	9	187